Overview M

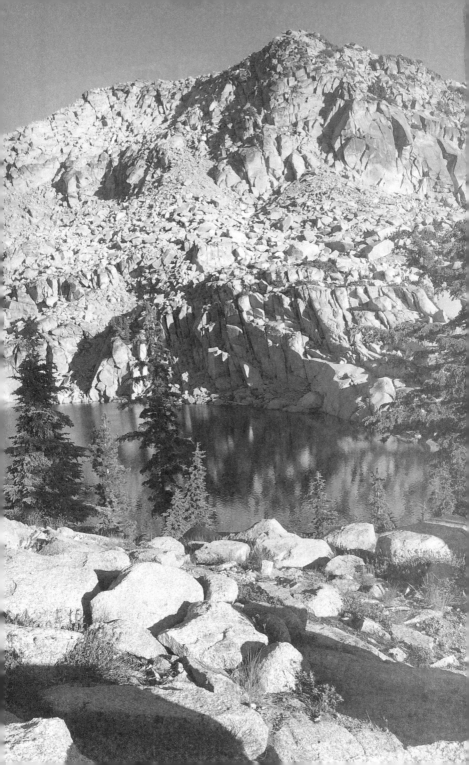

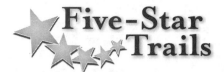

Five-Star
Trails

Lake Tahoe

40 Unforgettable Hikes in the Central Sierra Nevada

2ND EDITION

Jordan Summers

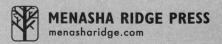

MENASHA RIDGE PRESS
menasharidge.com

Five-Star Trails: Lake Tahoe

Copyright © 2016 by Jordan Summers
All rights reserved
Published by Menasha Ridge Press
Printed in the United States of America
Distributed by Publishers Group West
Second edition, first printing

Project editor: Ritchey Halphen
Cover design: Scott McGrew
Cartography: Scott McGrew, Tony Hertzel, and Jordan Summers
Text design: Annie Long; typesetting and layout: Michele Myatt Quinn
Cover and interior photos: Jordan Summers, except where noted
Copyeditor: Kate McWhorter Johnson
Proofreaders: Laura Franck, L. Amanda Owens, Vanessa Lynn Rusch
Indexer: Sylvia Coates

Frontispiece: Desolation Wilderness is filled with inviting alpine tarns such as Smith Lake. *(See Hike 26, page 183.)*

Library of Congress Cataloging-in-Publication Data

Names: Summers, Jordan, 1951–
Title: Five-Star Trails: Lake Tahoe : 40 unforgettable hikes in the Central
    Sierra Nevada / Jordan Summers.
Description: Second edition. | Birmingham, AL : Menasha Ridge Press, [2016]
    Series: Five-Star Trails | "Distributed by Publishers Group West"—T.p.verso.
Identifiers: LCCN 2016019073 | ISBN 9781634040327 (paperback)
    ISBN 9781634040334 (e-book)
Subjects: LCSH: Hiking—Tahoe, Lake, Region (Calif. and Nev.)—Guidebooks.
    Tahoe, Lake (Calif. and Nev.)—Guidebooks.
Classification: LCC GV199.42.T16 S87 2016 | DDC 796.5109794/38—dc23
LC record available at lccn.loc.gov/2016019073

 MENASHA RIDGE PRESS
An imprint of AdventureKEEN
2204 First Ave. S., Suite 102
Birmingham, AL 35233
800-443-7227, fax 205-326-1012

Visit menasharidge.com for a complete listing of our books and for ordering information. Contact us at our website, at facebook.com/menasharidge, or at twitter.com/menasharidge with questions or comments. To find out more about who we are and what we're doing, visit blog.menasharidge.com.

Disclaimer This book is meant only as a guide to select trails in and around Lake Tahoe in California and Nevada and does not guarantee hiker safety in any way—you hike at your own risk. Neither Menasha Ridge Press nor Jordan Summers is liable for property loss or damage, personal injury, or death that may result from accessing or hiking the trails described in this guide. Be especially cautious when walking in potentially hazardous terrains with, for example, steep inclines or drop-offs. Do not attempt to explore terrain that may be beyond your abilities. Please read carefully the introduction to this book, as well as safety information from other sources. Familiarize yourself with current weather reports and maps of the area you plan to visit (in addition to the maps provided in this guidebook). Be aware of park regulations, and always follow them. While every effort has been made to ensure the accuracy of the information in this guidebook, land and road conditions, phone numbers and websites, and other information is subject to change.

Contents

Dedication

These beautiful hikes are dedicated to Taylor, Deacon, Finn, and Hunter.

Acknowledgments

MANY PEOPLE ARE RESPONSIBLE for the production of this guidebook. I am grateful to Molly Merkle at Menasha Ridge Press for her valuable support and guidance. I'm also thankful for the editing, cartography, design, and general project-nursing managed by Ritchey Halphen and aided by Annie Long, Scott McGrew, Kate Johnson, Laura Franck, Amanda Owens, and Vanessa Rusch.

Thanks to the many fellow hikers who told me about their favorite trails, described wildflower blooms, shared maps with me, snapped photos, and helped me identify flowers. I owe a big thanks to Eric Nichols for the many times he hiked Pyramid with me, winter, summer, and fall. And thanks as well for the many winter hikes we undertook in the Desolation and Mokelumne Wildernesses—in winds, on snow, over icy lakes, Eric went right along with me.

One casual trailhead conversation became my favorite hike: the Glen Alpine Loop, which Bill Bertram was kind enough to map out for me. Thanks to Raymond Morales and Emily Bullock, who first led me to the top of my favorite summit, Pyramid Peak. Emily coaxed me to the top when I was flat out of gas. And thanks to Wayne and Cindy McClelland, who not only clued me in to the trails and history around Incline Village but also guided me on the Folsom Camp Loop and coached me about the trail to Diamond Peak.

I'm grateful to the staff and volunteers of the Pacific Crest Trail Association for their continuous efforts to improve and maintain trails in the remote areas of the Lake Tahoe region. No less credit is due the Tahoe Rim Trail Association (TRTA) for its ambitious and fruitful efforts to create an environment that invites public use yet manages to lessen the negative impacts on both trails and lake.

Thanks to the TRTA's Justine Lentz and Lindsey Schultz, who each ensure that the trail is in superb condition and available to hikers through the association's many programs. I have to add that when I was bivied near their backcountry trail camp (in readiness for an early hike), they generously allowed me to join them for meals and refreshments.

Whether professional, seasonal, or volunteer, the hard work performed by trail crews benefits every hiker in the backcountry. Not only do they pour their sweat into the job, but they also know the trails intimately. Kudos to the generous volunteers who do this hard work on the Pacific Crest Trail and Tahoe Rim Trail.

The award for patience goes to my partner, Karin, who has waited at distant trailheads—Squaw Valley, Kingsbury South, Echo Lake, Ward Creek, Echo Summit—while I moseyed along watching clouds and taking pictures. And I met several fellow hikers who ferried me back to my car and helped me accomplish that act with some dignity.

It was only through the help of others, known and unknown alike, that I was able to accomplish the hikes and descriptions in this guidebook. I am grateful to you all.

—J. S.

Preface

I LIVE IN THE SACRAMENTO AREA, smack in the middle of the Central Valley—flat land just a few dozen feet above sea level. I make my weekly trips to Echo Summit or Incline Village and gasp for the fresh air as my lungs adjust to the elevation before I meander along my favorite trails. That's the routine during the no-snow season. During snow season, I keep at it along the foothill trails surrounding the Yuba and American Rivers. But the trails and destinations around Lake Tahoe are special compared with every other mountain locale's.

Look what happened in this one area of California. Ancient seafloors rose along with their altered sediments to become mountains. Molten rock from beneath the crust rose and cooled to form domes, peaks, and escarpments. Volcanoes released their molten innards across the landscape, covering it with ashfall, mudflows, or lava. And the valleys, cirques, tarns, and moraines scattered across this Sierra landscape are gifts of flowing rivers of ice. This is one incredible place because evidence of all this geologic activity is so easily visible. We see it today as Fallen Leaf Lake, the Crystal Range, Rockbound Valley, Mount Rose, Thunder Mountain, Velma Lakes, Half Moon Lake, Slide Mountain, and so on.

It is a hiker's great fortune that three renowned long trails converge in the Lake Tahoe vicinity. The famous Tahoe–Yosemite Trail originates here; the 165-mile Tahoe Rim Trail circumnavigates the lake on a backcountry route; and the crown jewel of long trails, the Pacific Crest Trail, merges at times with both of these famous tracks as its course runs north to south on the west side of Lake Tahoe. Compared to other trails in the backcountry, these three are the finest hikers can expect. These premier trails are graded, engineered, and signed for the benefit of hikers (and equestrians, officially).

I can't deny an urge to escape from the city in search of solitude in the mountains. That's a motivator for me, true. But I like to see other hikers getting out, enjoying the same backcountry that I'm able to enjoy. So I have a subtle motivation to share what I've experienced or to inform others how they can also have that experience. I hiked these trails at different times of the year, so you may not see exactly what I saw. But if I show you some identifiable signs along the way, you should have no trouble following along regardless of whether it's early, middle, or late season.

Despite 2014 and 2015 being low-snow, drought-stricken years, the snow we did have held on, and many of the trailheads were closed until the first week of June. Each spring, melting snow and warm days bring an explosion of color as flowers fly out of the ground, and hikers have so many options for where to go. I went hiking to Winnemucca Lake during an absolute riot of color and perfumed scents. Name the plant and it was there. And do butterflies like nectar? From the peaks to the meadows, these flying flowers were swarming in massive droves whenever I encountered them. Pick a creek and flowers will line it; from forested Lyons Creek to granite-bound Silver Creek, flowers find a way to fill every crack and crevice.

Most years, I could safely predict a thunderstorm by 3 in the afternoon, every afternoon. This year, the rain stayed away, but the lightning came in its place, threatening a wildland blaze but never any quenching relief for the drought. A brief splatter here and there, sometimes a clamorous hailstorm, but no soil-soaking gully washers.

In identifying and describing flora and fauna, I attempted to check myself and leave my lowland brain in the foothills. I expect to hear about it if I identified a Jeffrey pine as its foothill twin, the ponderosa pine. The same applies to incense cedars and Western junipers. (Where did I put my glasses?)

This edition includes the actual Thunder Mountain, which I was glad to finally identify correctly. This year, I was held back from summiting Pyramid Peak due to winds that moved me around at will. It's pretty easy to ascend with normal care, but the gusts were just too dangerous this time. The next day's hike up Ralston Peak was as mild as could be. The views from Mount Tallac were as wonderful as ever, but those from Twin Peaks eluded my gaze again when one of the rare sprinkles made it wet enough for me to feel unsure of ascending the summit on wet rock. And a pounding hailstorm with wicked lightning sent me scurrying back downhill, ending my track 250 feet before touching Jabu Lake on a side trip from LeConte.

I will unabashedly confess that there have been more than a few times that found me so interested in the surroundings—scenery near and far, flowers, trees, bear scat—that I have walked into trees, missed junctions, bashed into small boulders, backtracked, returned, and rehiked. All normally embarrassing actions, but none seem to bother me in the Tahoe backcountry. If you miss a trail or pass a junction, I hope this guide gives you enough information to happily continue on your new adventure.

My sincere goal is that you'll find a hike or destination in this book that will interest you, that this book will guide you there and return you safely, and that your good hike will encourage you to invite others for a similar experience.

To paraphrase George Wharton James from his 1915 descriptive account, *The Lake of the Sky:* Get out!

—*Jordan Summers*
Elk Grove, California

Recommended Hikes

Scenic Hikes

The entire Table of Contents could go here—every one of these hikes is incredibly scenic.

Most Difficult Hikes

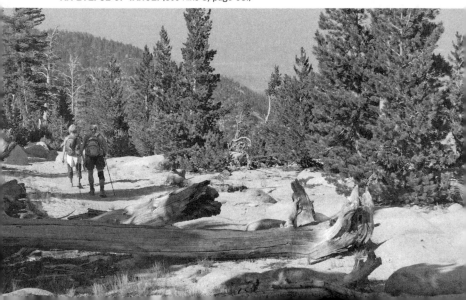

HIKERS PASSING FREEL PEAK ON THE TAHOE RIM TRAIL ARE ABOUT TO GET AN EYEFUL OF TAHOE. *(See Hike 8, page 68.)*

Easiest Hikes

Best for Solitude

Good for Children

Best for Wildflowers

As is the case for the Scenic Hikes, all 40 hikes offer wonderful displays of wildflowers.

Best for Birding

Steepest Hikes

Hikes Requiring Permits

Flattest Hikes

Scrambling Hikes

Wheelchair-Accessible Hikes

Best for Dogs

Hikes by Category

Day Loops

Day Out-and-Backs

Day Out-and-Backs *(continued)*

Day Shuttles

Overnight Loops

Overnight Out-and-Backs

Overnight Shuttles

Hikes Less Than 6 Miles

Hikes 6–10 Miles

Hikes More Than 10 Miles

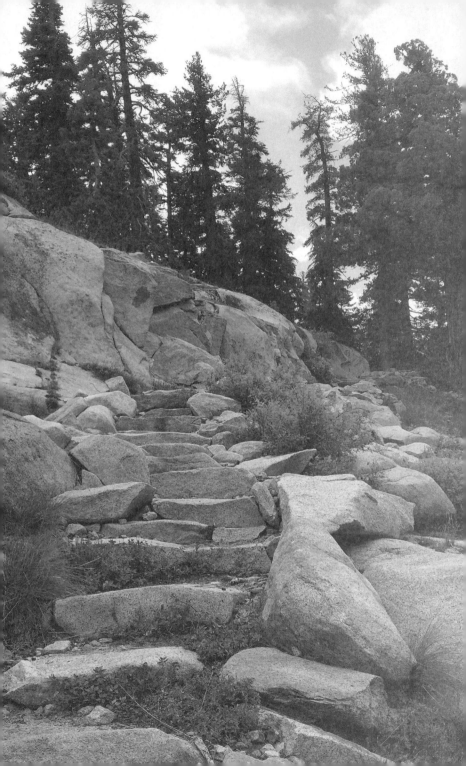

Introduction

About This Book

THE LAKE TAHOE REGION is a magnet for outdoor enthusiasts, who are drawn there by the millions. Despite the abundance of lofty superlatives that inevitably precede a visit, Lake Tahoe's descriptions do not seem to disappoint anyone.

More than 125 trails are in active use around the Tahoe Basin, and several of the 40 hikes described in these pages represent the region's most popular destinations. Other hikes lead away from the crowds and often take a more difficult route. Trails and destinations are so plentiful in the central Sierra Nevada that these hikes are restricted to an area within 25 miles of the lake's shore.

In the 1840s, explorer John C. Fremont described Lake Tahoe as a mountain lake so entirely surrounded by mountains that he could not discover an outlet (although the Washoe Indians had drawn him a map three years earlier). He mapped the area and called the lake, yes, Mountain Lake. (Why was he an engineer, you ask, when he had such a command of the language?) More-poetic heads eventually prevailed: By 1870 it was settled, after ousting a sullied governor's moniker, that the Washoe Indian words for "big water"—*tah-oo*— would be a proper name for the spectacular lake. Afterward, it was just a matter of agreeing on its pronunciation.

Fremont was no quitter, but he missed the lake's only outlet, which is located on its western shore. It's where Tahoe City stands today and where the Truckee River has most often originated when not blocked by ice dams. The current lake level is 6,228 feet, and the Rubicon Trail comes closest to that mark in this book. Freel Peak in California and Nevada's Mount Rose are the geographic high points

IMPROVEMENTS SUCH AS STAIRS ARE OFTEN DEVELOPED BY VOLUNTEERS.

around the lake. Both summits are least 4,500 feet above the waves and are among the peaks that you can reach following these notes.

Lake Tahoe's history is brief but by no means uneventful. Within a decade of Fremont's mapping of it, gold was discovered and exploited in the foothills, and California had become a state. Subsequently, silver was discovered in adjacent Nevada, and the settlement and economic exploitation of Lake Tahoe's natural resources went unabated. Today, great emphasis is placed on preserving the natural resources and creating diverse outdoor recreation opportunities.

Many of the notes herein refer to geologic processes and geographic features. You'll find clear explanations of these in geology and natural-history guides and texts, which are referenced in Appendix D. If you don't have those available, this simple explainer might suffice: The mountains around Lake Tahoe are a mess. They are a jumble of pieces from several puzzles—and you can see the types of pieces on each of these hikes. No skills necessary.

Basically, Nevada used to border (approximately) the Pacific Ocean. Then, beginning a few hundred million years ago, a chunk of land similar in size and shape to Japan slammed into that beach. *Voilà,* new property. New mountains were also formed because the land kept coming. It scrunched up the former beaches and slid under older property. This happened two more times. Each event was followed by lots of volcanoes along the line of the new property. Starting about 250 million years ago, some of the earth's crust melted and rose in the form of large granite blobs that are now called batholiths. This happened from time to time over the next 150 million years. Less than 50 million years ago, the Sierra Nevada started uplifting from the west. This uplift set off the erosive force of water, and river channels were cut into the terrain. More volcanoes grew along the old coast, and their ash, lava, and mudflows covered much of the original terrain. This went on in such volume for so long that Sierran rivers were filled, passes were covered, and terrain buried. Simple erosion took care of most of that soft volcanic material, and the rivers reestablished themselves.

Then, about 1.5 million years ago, the cleanup crew showed up in the form of ice. Glaciers formed, covering peaks less than 13,000 feet high with a cap of ice stretching from Lake Tahoe to Yosemite. The erosive grinding power of the glaciers scraped away much of the debris, sometimes forming it into nice, neat piles that we call moraines. Most of the granite was eroded not by the ice itself but by the subsequent freeze–thaw action of water, which causes the granite to wear away by cracking or exfoliating, and the process continues with each annual cycle. *Et voici!* (as François Matthes might have said), you have a considerable jumble of rocks to play on.

The hikes in this guidebook take you all over that playground, leading to tarns, cirques, moraines, and horns. These hikes don't require you to climb mountains to enjoy being on mountains. Some hikes are connected to other hikes or can be readjusted to create a shorter or longer trek. Most hikes visit lakes, streams, meadows, or peaks, all of which are created by natural processes that are often interconnected, such as the succession meadow that grows at McConnell Lake or the soil building on Tallac's scree slopes. A natural-history guide in your pack will help make these processes come alive on the trail.

Use the overview map and regional maps to find possibilities for creating your own custom hikes. I approached several of these hikes in that manner to create interesting and rewarding treks. Hikers can do many things to increase their enjoyment of the hikes on the following pages. Enter the trailhead waypoints into Google Earth or other mapping software, and look for trails in the vicinity. It's not unusual that one trailhead serves as the embarkation point for several hikes.

How to Use This Guidebook

The following section walks you through this book's organization, making it easy and convenient to plan great hikes.

The Overview Map, Overview Map Key, and Legend

The overview map on the inside front cover shows the primary trailheads for all 40 hikes. The numbers on the overview map pair with the map key on the facing page. A legend explaining the map symbols used throughout the book appears on the inside back cover.

Regional Maps

This book is divided into regions, and prefacing each regional chapter is an overview map. The regional maps provide more detail than the overview map, bringing you closer to the hikes.

Trail Maps

In addition to the overview map and regional maps, a detailed map of each hike's route appears with its profile. On each of these maps, symbols indicate the trailhead, the complete route, significant features, facilities, and topographic landmarks such as creeks, overlooks, and peaks.

To produce the highly accurate maps in this book, I used a handheld GPS unit to gather data while hiking each route, then sent that data to Menasha Ridge Press's expert cartographers. Be aware, though, that your GPS device is no substitute for sound, sensible navigation that takes into account the conditions that you observe while hiking.

Elevation Profile

Each hike includes this graphical element in addition to a trail map. Each entry's key information also lists the elevation at the trailhead and at the hike's high point.

The elevation diagram represents the rises and falls of the trail as viewed from the side, over the complete distance (in miles) of that trail. On the diagram's vertical axis, or height scale, the number of feet indicated between each tick mark lets you visualize the climb. To avoid making flat hikes look steep and steep hikes appear flat, varying height scales provide an accurate image of each hike's climbing challenge.

The Hike Profile

This book contains a concise and informative narrative that describes each hike from beginning to end. The text will get you from a well-known road or highway to the trailhead, through the twists and turns of the hike route, and back to the trailhead.

At the beginning of each hike's full description are its star ratings and at-a-glance information. A sample from Hike 25, Sylvia and Lyon Lakes (page 178), follows, with an explanation of each element:

STAR RATINGS

The hikes in *Five-Star Trails: Lake Tahoe* were carefully chosen to give the hiker a stellar experience overall and represent the diversity of trails found in the region. Each hike was assigned a one- to five-star rating in each of the following categories: scenery, trail condition, suitability for children, level of difficulty, and degree of solitude. Here's how the star ratings for each of the five categories break down:

FOR SCENERY:

★ ★ ★ ★ ★	Unique, picturesque panoramas
★ ★ ★ ★	Diverse vistas
★ ★ ★	Pleasant views
★ ★	Unchanging landscape
★	Not selected for scenery

FOR TRAIL CONDITION:

★ ★ ★ ★ ★	Consistently well maintained
★ ★ ★ ★	Stable, with no surprises
★ ★ ★	Average terrain to negotiate
★ ★	Inconsistent, with good and poor areas
★	Rocky, overgrown, or often muddy

FOR CHILDREN:

★ ★ ★ ★ ★	Babes in strollers are welcome
★ ★ ★ ★	Fun for any kid past the toddler stage
★ ★ ★	Good for young hikers with proven stamina
★ ★	Not enjoyable for children
★	Not advisable for children

(continued on page 7)

Sample Profile:
Sylvia and Lyons Lakes

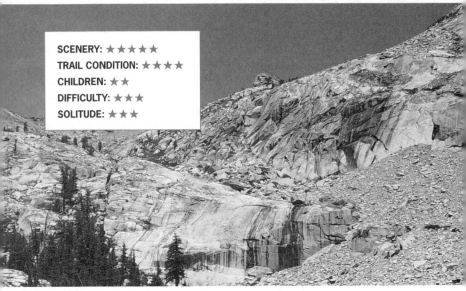

SCENERY: ★★★★★
TRAIL CONDITION: ★★★★
CHILDREN: ★★
DIFFICULTY: ★★★
SOLITUDE: ★★

LYONS LAKE STANDS SENTINEL ON THE SOUTH SIDE OF THE CRYSTAL RANGE.

GPS TRAILHEAD COORDINATES: N38° 48.626′ W120° 14.367′

DISTANCE & CONFIGURATION: 12-mile out-and-back

HIKING TIME: 6 hours

OUTSTANDING FEATURES: Massive granite wall at north end of Lyons Lake; shallow pools along the steps of Lyons Creek; base camp beneath Pyramid Peak

ELEVATION: 6,730′ at trailhead

ACCESS: Depends on snow; permits required for day hiking and overnight camping. Pick up your free day permit at the kiosk adjacent to the trailhead, which is marked by a green gate. Overnight camping permits are available for a fee at the Taylor Creek Visitor Center, 150 yards to the west of Fallen Leaf Lake Road on CA 89, or online at tinyurl.com/dwovernightcamping.

MAP: *Desolation Wilderness* (Wilderness Press)

FACILITIES: Pit toilet

COMMENTS: Bring sunglasses and sunscreen.

CONTACT: US Forest Service, Taylor Creek Visitor Center, 530-543-2674, tinyurl.com/taylorcreekvisitorcenter

(continued from page 5)

FOR DIFFICULTY:

★ ★ ★ ★ ★	Grueling
★ ★ ★ ★	Challenging, with stretches of ease
★ ★ ★	Exhilarating
★ ★	Pleasantly invigorating
★	Good for a relaxing stroll

FOR SOLITUDE:

★ ★ ★ ★ ★	Positively tranquil
★ ★ ★ ★	Spurts of isolation
★ ★ ★	Moderately secluded
★ ★	Crowded on weekends and holidays
★	Steady stream of individuals and/or groups

GPS TRAILHEAD COORDINATES

As noted in "Trail Maps," page 4, I used a handheld GPS unit to obtain geographic data and sent the information to Menasha Ridge's cartographers. In the at-a-glance information for each hike profile, I've provided the intersection of the latitude (north) and longitude (west) coordinates to orient you at the trailhead. In some cases, you can drive within viewing distance of a trailhead. Other hikes require a short walk to reach the trailhead from a parking area. Either way, the coordinates are given from the trail's actual head—its point of origin.

This guidebook expresses GPS coordinates in degree–decimal minute format. The latitude–longitude grid system is likely quite familiar to you, but here's a refresher, pertinent to visualizing the coordinates:

Imaginary lines of latitude—called *parallels* and approximately 69 miles apart from each other—run horizontally around the globe. The equator is established to be 0°, and each parallel is indicated by degrees from the equator: up to 90°N at the North Pole and down to 90°S at the South Pole.

Imaginary lines of longitude—called *meridians*—run perpendicular to latitude lines. Longitude lines are likewise indicated by degrees. Starting from 0° at the Prime Meridian in Greenwich, England, they continue to the east and west until they meet 180° later at the International Date Line in the Pacific Ocean. At the equator, longitude lines also are approximately 69 miles apart, but that distance narrows as the meridians converge toward the North and South Poles.

To convert GPS coordinates in degrees, minutes, and seconds to degrees–decimal minutes, the seconds are divided by 60. For more on GPS technology, visit usgs.gov.

DISTANCE AND CONFIGURATION

"Distance" notes the length of the hike round-trip, from start to finish. If the hike description includes options to shorten or extend the hike, those round-trip distances are also included here. "Configuration" defines the type of route—for example, a loop, an out-and-back (which takes you in and out the same way), or a shuttle (one-way route).

HIKING TIME

Two miles per hour is a general rule of thumb for the hiking times noted in this guidebook. That pace typically allows time for taking photos, for dawdling and admiring views, and for alternating stretches of hills and descents. When deciding whether or not to follow a particular trail in this guidebook, consider the weather, plus your own pace, general physical condition, and energy level on a given day.

HIKERS WIND ACROSS BIG MEADOW ON FLOWER-FILLED TAHOE RIM TRAIL TO DARDANELLES AND ROUND LAKES AND THEN CARSON PASS.

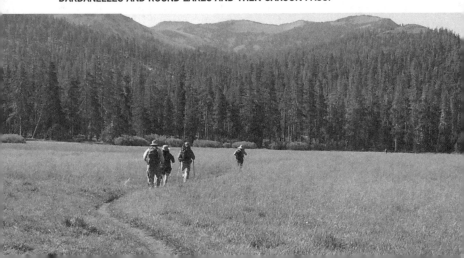

OUTSTANDING FEATURES

Lists highlights that draw hikers to the trail: mountain or forest views, water features, historic sites, and the like.

ELEVATION

The at-a-glance information includes the elevation at the trailhead. The full hike profile also includes a complete elevation profile (see page 4).

ACCESS

Lists when the trail is open; also notes (if applicable) whether any fees or permits are required to hike the trail.

MAPS

Resources for maps, in addition to those in this guidebook, are listed here. As noted earlier, we recommend that you carry more than one map—and that you consult those maps before heading out on the trail.

FACILITIES

Includes visitor centers, restrooms, water, picnic tables, and other basics at or near the trailhead.

COMMENTS

Here, you'll find assorted nuggets of information, such as whether or not dogs are allowed on the trails. Note that not every hike has this listing.

CONTACTS

Listed here are phone numbers and websites for checking trail conditions, trail-access hours and seasons, and other day-to-day information before you head out.

Overview, Route Details, and Directions

These four elements compose the heart of the hike. "Overview" gives you a quick summary of what to expect on that trail; "Route Details" guides you on the hike, from start to finish; and "Directions" will get you to the trailhead from a well-known road or highway.

Climate

Lake Tahoe displays some climatic variety near each of the cardinal points around the region—South Lake Tahoe has different weather from that in Tahoe City, which is different from the weather in Truckee or Incline Village. But it really boils down to the activities that you can undertake around the lake. Lake Tahoe's weather is either sunny with snow on the ground or sunny with no snow on the ground.

Tahoe seems to have two distinct seasons. First there's snow season, and then there's hiking, biking, climbing, and anything-else-that-doesn't-need-snow season. Typically beginning in mid-May, the spring–summer–fall season lasts about five months or until the first snows in early November. The snowpack lingers in the Tahoe area later into spring due to the unique pattern of high daytime temperatures followed by freezing temperatures at night. However, spring opens hastily with dozens of plant species eager to get up and get busy. Summer morphs into autumn without notice as every area begins to dry out after having put on an outstanding colorful display. The one type of summertime display that hikers need to avoid is lightning. Just about every afternoon, the sky brews up a threatening batch of clouds—an atmospheric caution flag to anyone approaching a peak, ridge, or exposed rocky area.

Lake Tahoe gets its moisture-laden air from the same place it gets its weekend visitors: from the San Francisco Bay Area. Prevailing westerly winds carry moisture right up to Donner Pass and Echo Summit as they blow eastward along the watershed canyons of the Yuba and American rivers. These warm valley winds rise as they run directly into the Sierra Nevada, which blocks their paths. The average annual snowfall of 2 feet in Colfax is eclipsed 46 miles away by that of Donner Summit's 34 feet.

Before every drive to Lake Tahoe to "conduct research," I checked and rechecked the National Weather Service forecasts at the National Oceanographic and Atmospheric Administration's website,

Lake Tahoe Climate (at Tahoe City, California)

MONTH	RAINFALL		SNOWFALL		AVG HIGH		AVG LOW	
	in	cm	in	cm	°F	°C	°F	°C
Jan	6.18	16	43.8	111	36	2	16	−9
Feb	5.50	14	38.0	97	39	4	18	−8
Mar	4.11	10	35.5	90	44	7	21	−6
Apr	2.11	5.4	15.2	39	50	10	26	−3
May	1.19	3.0	3.8	10	60	16	32	0
June	0.69	1.8	0.2	0.5	69	21	37	3
July	0.26	0.7	0.0	0.0	79	26	43	6
Aug	0.31	0.8	0.0	0.0	78	26	42	6
Sept	0.64	1.6	0.3	0.8	70	21	37	3
Oct	1.83	4.6	2.4	6.1	51	11	31	−1
Nov	3.68	9.3	16.2	41	47	8	24	−4
Dec	5.40	14	33.5	85	40	4	20	−7

noaa.gov/weather. This is an essential step in preparing for any day or overnight hike.

Water

You would think this wouldn't be a topic of caution, what with some three-and-a-half-gazillion crystal-clear gallons of it captured in Lake Tahoe. But water is an issue in the Lake Tahoe region just as it is everywhere—possibly more so, in fact. Most local bumpers carry a sticker entreating everyone to "Keep Tahoe Blue." Trails around here have been designed or reengineered to specifically abate the effect of runoff water, which can carry huge loads of sediment into the lake.

Few hikes in this guidebook don't come near or cross water in some form. And that water is especially important for hikers, for both recreation and hydration. Throughout these chapters, I have suggested possible fill-up spots for you and your water system (bottles or bags). During periods of drought, many streams flow with less volume, disappear earlier in the season, or are entirely nonexistent throughout the summer. Hikers are strongly advised to carry water as if they would encounter none on the trail.

Giardia lamblia remains a persistent problem in this region as in all other backcountry areas. Since cattle are no longer prevalent, wildlife biologists have noted a downturn in the levels of this pathogen, but it remains at dangerous levels due to the impact of humans and the animals they bring with them. *Hint:* If you've been following hoof prints or paw prints, you may want to watch where you get water. Chances are that the maker of the prints got water there, too.

For this reason, I strongly caution that all water is suspect, regardless of its clarity. (My microscopic eyesight has diminished slightly, so I can't see the bad guys anyway.) There are a few reliable methods of water treatment specific to giardia and cryptosporidium. Filtering works, as do chlorine dioxide tablets, iodine tablets, chemical mixes, and UV light. In camp, water can be purified by bringing the water to a boil—at the first bubble, it's pure. Just pick the method that suits you for both convenience and taste, and then rigorously use it on any drinking water in the backcountry.

All of these methods work, but they must be used in order to be effective. This is important. A case of giardiasis is not pleasant, and getting it takes just one drink from that "crystal-clear stream."

Clothing

It should be as simple as throwing on a pair of trail runners and a pair of shorts, which is fine, but there are risks to that approach. These risks span from merely not enjoying the hike on the not-so-problematic end all the way to "death will come within four hours" on the other end.

Some well-chosen duds can mean the difference between a pleasant trip and a dismal search-and-rescue-team after-action report.

- ★ **KILLER COTTON.** The Fatal Fabric. These are names for that fabric that is oh-so-comfortable on a hot summer day but lethal when worn in the backcountry. Eliminate it from your hiking closet and use synthetics, silk, or wool for your body-covering needs.

- ★ **BASE LAYER.** This layer is responsible for wicking moisture, that is, perspiration, away from your skin so that it can evaporate without cooling your skin. Undershorts and a shirt of wicking material will keep you dry and warm. Cotton feels great next to your skin until it becomes sweat-soaked.

- ★ **INSULATION LAYER.** A wicking T-shirt isn't enough to insulate your body when the temperatures drop or the wind picks up. A layer of a synthetic fleece or a wool sweater will help hold warm air around your body. Another protective layer, such as a wind jacket, can be used effectively. A soft-shell garment often provides not only insulation but also water and wind repellency.

- ★ **OUTER LAYER.** Quick-drying, durable shorts or convertible pants with lots of pockets are standard trail outerwear. A lightweight long-sleeved shirt will offer some sun protection on long, exposed stretches, and a lightweight wind shirt can guard against warmth-robbing breezes.

- ★ **SOFT-SHELL JACKET.** Coated with a durable water- and wind-repelling finish, this garment can ward off light rain and also insulate, depending on the lining thickness.

- ★ **RAINGEAR.** This clothing should shed rain on the outside and allow you to remain dry on the inside. A hooded jacket or an anorak (one zips and one pulls over your head) should have pit zips for ventilation. Pants should have zippered cuffs so you can easily put them on and take them off.

- ★ **BANDANA.** Like a clothing multitool, it's great for swatting at mosquitoes, wiping brows, and acting as an impromptu hat.

- ★ **BOOTS.** Lightweight hiking boots rather than trail shoes are my recommendation for every natural trail.

- ★ **GAITERS.** This accessory is almost essential for me to keep dirt, sticks, seeds, and other crud from getting inside my boots and the burrs off my socks.

Essential Gear

What I decide to carry with me on every outing depends in large part on where I'm headed and what I'll be doing there: a minimum for day hikes, mostly the same plus food and a stove for overnight, more food and more person-patching supplies for longer treks. The clothing, sleeping bag, and shelter vary depending on conditions.

These are the essentials that I carry on every hike in the mountains. Some items I hope I'll never use. The emergency-only items can, however, prevent a simple injury from turning into a life-threatening ordeal. Because I hike solo and I'm unable to predict the outcome of every hike, I prepare to some extent by asking myself, "Which emergency *won't* happen to me on this trip?"

So I don't have to worry about memorizing a long list of items, I use these *-tion* ("shun") words to describe essential gear.

- ★ **PREPARATION:** A plan of your route, your gear, your destination, and your return time to be left with an emergency contact, along with instructions for what to do in case the return time is missed

- ★ **NAVIGATION:** The route description, a trail or topographic map, a simple compass, and the knowledge to use them (a GPS receiver or altimeter for increased precision and speed)

- ★ **HYDRATION:** Full water reservoirs, plus extra; water-treatment tablets or purifying filter

- ★ **NUTRITION:** Nutrition bars, snacks, or meals for the day plus extra

- ★ **IGNITION:** Matches, lighter, or other fire starter, plus stove with full fuel bottle or canister

- ★ **ILLUMINATION:** Headlamp with *fresh* batteries

- ★ **RADIATION:** Sun hat, sunglasses, sunscreen, lip balm, UV-resistant clothes

- ★ **INSULATION:** Base layer (wicking), insulation layer, rain gear, extra socks, soft-shell jacket, extra (unworn) insulating garment

- ★ **MEDICATION:** Your personal daily medicines, plus first-aid kit with fresh supplies, instructions, and the knowledge to use them

★ **PROTECTION:** Space blanket, tarp (to shelter accident victims in sun or rain), survival bivy sack (to warm victims of hypothermia, including yourself)

★ **STABILIZATION:** Trekking poles (third leg, monopod, shelter pole, cougar and bear defense, poison oak deflector, general poking and irritating of small creatures)

★ **IN ADDITION:** Emergency-contact list, signal whistle, signal mirror, knife, multitool, cord

Additional Gear

For day hikes I use a 33- to 45-liter pack, for overnight hikes I carry a 45- to 48-liter pack, and for longer hikes I carry a 58- or 60-liter pack. Aside from the essential gear that I carry on every hike in the mountains, I carry a few extra things—packing as light as possible—that might help make your hikes more enjoyable, too.

★ Camera

★ Extra batteries

★ Field guides

★ GPS device

★ Mini-tripod

★ "Monocular" (half of a pair of binoculars)

★ Notebook and pencil

★ Specimen bags

★ Trowel and hygiene kit

Overnight hikes don't require much more gear. I use various one-man tents and bivy systems.

★ Camp shoes

★ Down sweater

★ Food (1.5 pounds per person, per day)

★ Sleeping bag (rated to 30°)

★ Stove, fuel, and pot with lid

★ Tent or bivy with groundsheet

Without being overly precise about it, the total of my gear for a three-day hike would not exceed 35 pounds. On the other hand, my day pack was never less than 23 pounds. Your needs certainly will vary.

First-Aid Kit

A typical first-aid kit may contain more items than you might think necessary. These are just the basics. Prepackaged kits in waterproof bags (Atwater Carey and Adventure Medical make a variety of kits) are available. Even though quite a few items are listed here, they pack down into a small space:

★ Antibacterial wound-cleansing wipes and ointment (such as Neosporin)

★ Aspirin, acetaminophen (Tylenol), or ibuprofen (Advil)

★ Athletic tape

★ Blister kit (moleskin or an adhesive variety such as Spenco 2nd Skin)

★ Butterfly-closure bandages

★ Diphenhydramine (Benadryl), in case of allergic reactions

★ Elastic bandages (such as Ace) or joint wraps (such as Spenco)

★ Epinephrine in a prefilled syringe (EpiPen), typically by prescription only, for people known to have severe allergic reactions to hiking mishaps such as bee stings

★ Gauze (one roll and a half-dozen 4-by-4-inch pads)

★ Hydrogen peroxide or iodine

★ Insect repellent

General Safety

To some potential mountain enthusiasts, the deep woods seem inordinately dark and perilous. It's the fear of the unknown that causes this anxiety. No doubt, potentially dangerous situations can occur outdoors, but as long as you use sound judgment and prepare yourself before hitting the trail, you'll be much safer in the woods than in most urban areas of the country. It's better to look at a backcountry hike as a fascinating chance to discover the unknown rather than a chance for potential disaster. If you're new to the game, I suggest starting out easy and finding a person who knows more to help you out. In addition, here are a few tips to make your trip safer and easier.

★ **ALWAYS CARRY FOOD AND WATER,** whether you're planning to go overnight or not. Food will give you energy, help keep you warm, and sustain you in an emergency until help arrives. You never know if you'll have a stream nearby when you become thirsty. Bring potable water or treat water before drinking it from a stream. Boil or filter all found water before drinking it.

★ **STAY ON DESIGNATED TRAILS.** Even on the most clearly marked trails, you usually reach a point where you have to stop and consider in which direction to head. If you become disoriented, don't panic. As soon as you think you may be off-track, stop, assess your current direction, and then retrace your steps to the point where you went astray. Using a map, a compass, and this book, and keeping in mind what you've passed thus far, reorient yourself and trust your judgment on which way to continue. If you become absolutely unsure of how to continue, return to your vehicle the way you came in. Should you become completely lost and have no idea how to find the trailhead, remaining in place along the trail and waiting for help is most often the best option for adults and always the best option for children.

★ **BE ESPECIALLY CAREFUL WHEN CROSSING STREAMS.** Whether you're fording the stream or crossing on a log, make every step count. If you have any doubt about maintaining your balance on a log, ford the stream instead: Use a trekking pole or stout stick for balance and *face upstream as you cross.* If a stream seems too deep to ford, turn back. Whatever is on the other side isn't worth risking your life for.

★ **BE CAREFUL AT OVERLOOKS.** While these areas may provide spectacular views, they are potentially hazardous. Stay back from the edge of outcrops, and make absolutely sure of your footing—a misstep can mean a nasty and possibly fatal fall.

★ **STANDING DEAD TREES** and storm-damaged living trees pose a real hazard to hikers and tent campers. These trees may have loose or broken limbs that could fall at any time. When choosing a spot to rest or a backcountry campsite, *look up.*

★ **KNOW THE SYMPTOMS OF SUBNORMAL BODY TEMPERATURE, OR HYPOTHERMIA.** Shivering and forgetfulness are the two most common indicators of this stealthy killer. Hypothermia can occur at any elevation, even in the summer, especially if you're wearing lightweight cotton clothing. If symptoms develop, get to shelter, hot liquids, and dry clothes or a sleeping bag as soon as possible.

★ **TAKE ALONG YOUR BRAIN.** A cool, calculating mind is the single most important asset on the trail. Think before you act. Watch your step. Plan ahead. Avoiding accidents before they happen is the best way to ensure a rewarding and relaxing hike.

★ **ASK QUESTIONS.** Public-land employees are there to help. It's a lot easier to solicit advice before a problem occurs, and it will help you avoid a mishap away from civilization when it's too late to amend an error.

Animal, Insect, and Plant Hazards

MOSQUITOES You will encounter mosquitoes on most of the hikes in this book. Insect repellent and/or repellent-impregnated clothing are the only simple methods to ward off these pests. Mosquitoes in California are known to carry West Nile virus, so all due caution should be taken to avoid mosquito bites.

BEES AND WASPS Unless you're allergic to the sting of bees or wasps, these insects should not be considered dangerous to you. Sit next to a batch of wildflowers—right up close—and watch the bees fly in and out as they maul the colorful buds. You're invisible to the bees, which are concentrating on far sweeter treats than you. Enjoy your hike without worrying about these helpful insects.

You may, however, have an opportunity to chance upon a wild hive while following any of these hikes. If you hear a constant buzzing that grows louder with your approach, walk away, as you have likely found a hive or a swarm. Bees will attack if their hive or queen is threatened.

TICKS A tick is a bloodsucking arachnid (related to spiders—not an insect) found in almost every outdoor environment, usually in low trees and tall grasses. Of the nine species of ticks found in

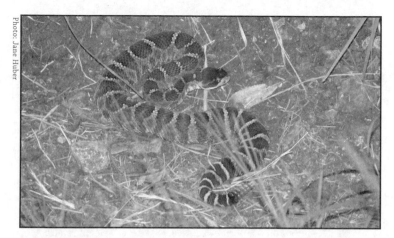

Photo: Jane Huber

RATTLESNAKE

California, the Western black-legged deer tick has been labeled as the vector for Lyme disease. Lyme disease has been reported in the Lake Tahoe region.

These tiny parasites are about the size of a freckle or sesame seed and are hard to stop from landing on your body. You can spray or wear repellent-impregnated clothing, but the best method for dealing with them is to conduct a thorough inspection of your entire body and then remove any ticks you find.

POISON OAK A concern that you can dismiss in these parts is a rash from poison oak. This three-leaved plant does not grow above 5,000 feet, so you won't encounter it in the Lake Tahoe region.

RATTLESNAKES Northern California's only native pit viper, the Northern Pacific rattlesnake, makes its home in the Sierra Nevada foothills, and its range extends to the Upper Montane Belt—approximately 5,000–7,500 feet in elevation in the northern range.

Mountain Lions
These big cats inhabit every corner of California and range over a 100-square-mile home territory. They are present wherever deer are

abundant. Also called the cougar, puma, or panther, the mountain lion is tan-coated, has black-tipped ears and tail, weighs up to 150 pounds, and is about 7 feet long from nose to tail. Cubs are invariably cute and covered with dark-brown spots.

Mountain lions are important to the natural community, and this is their home. They are seldom seen but have been known to attack humans without warning. Therefore, hikers need to be alert to their presence. Some advice:

★ **AVOID HIKING ALONE** at dawn or dusk, and closely supervise children. Cougars are drawn to children and dogs because their size and motions mimic those of their prey.

★ **NEVER APPROACH A MOUNTAIN LION.** If you hear or see a mountain lion, stay calm and don't scream. If you stumble upon an animal's corpse—whether fresh or rotting—depart the area immediately. This is probably a cougar's well-guarded meal.

★ **IF CONFRONTED BY A COUGAR,** do anything to make yourself appear larger: Raise your outspread arms, wave hiking sticks or tree limbs, gather other hikers (especially children) next to you. Act threatening, but allow the animal a path to escape. Absolutely avoid bending over or turning your back on a mountain lion, and *do not run*—cougars will interpret these actions as those of their prey. Make noise, use your firmest outside voice, and throw rocks at its body.

★ **TRY TO REMAIN STANDING IF YOU ARE ATTACKED,** because lions will try to bite the neck or head. Use any instrument at hand to repel the cat. *Always try to fight back.* In 2006, a woman successfully used a ballpoint pen to fight off the mountain lion that was attacking her husband. Both she and her husband survived.

California Black Bears

With the possible exception of mountain lions, most animals will be scared of you and won't pose a threat as long as you respect their space. Then there are black bears.

The Desolation Wilderness is the black bears' home. We can only visit.

California has a large population of black bears, which are actually cinnamon to dark brown in color. These bears are very intelligent and are always searching for large quantities of food to build their nutrition stores. Despite weighing up to 500 pounds, black bears can run up to 35 miles an hour. Herein lies the threat.

Most bears fear people and will leave when they see you. But if a bear woofs, snaps its jaws, slaps the ground or brush, or bluff-charges: *You're too close! Back away now! Don't take any pictures!*

Conflicts between bears and humans usually occur because bears want your food. It's easy pickings, after all. And if a bear can nab your food, it will nab someone else's. Thus, the bear becomes a nuisance bear. Nuisance bears are removed from the area once; then, if they return to forage on human food—and they will—they are destroyed.

So secure your food for the protection of yourself and the bears. Locate your camp kitchen away from your sleeping area, and keep the area free of food spills. It's also best if your backpack doesn't smell of trout and you don't store your candy supply in your tent.

Don't leave food out or unattended—even for a few minutes. Use a bear-proof canister to carry and store your food when backpacking. These canisters can be rented for free at the US Forest Service Visitor Center at Taylor Creek and the Lake Tahoe Basin Management Unit office (see Appendix A).

If a bear is eating your food or shredding your pack in search of your snacks, don't throw rocks at the bear's head or face, and *don't ever* attempt to retrieve any of your grub. In the bear's mind, it's now his food, so let him have it. This way, you can walk away with a great story. If you try to reclaim the food, you won't.

In the unlikely event that you do encounter a black bear on the trail, don't run. Make eye contact without staring. Pick up small children to keep them from running. Back away slowly. Stay calm and don't scream. Speak to the bear in your best outdoor voice.

If a bear approaches within about 75 feet, make yourself appear larger by spreading your arms, waving hiking sticks or branches, or holding your jacket open. Do not block the bear's escape route. Attacks are rare, but if a bear is after you and not your food, throw rocks and make every attempt to frighten it away or *fight it off aggressively* with anything at hand. Don't bother to run—as noted previously, black bears are very fast.

Backcountry Advice

When you enter the backcountry to camp or day-hike (with the proper permit, of course—see Appendix B), it's a help to other hikers, the environment, and yourself to adhere to the adages "Pack it in, pack it out" and "Take only pictures, leave only footprints." Practicing Leave No Trace ethics in the backcountry benefits everyone.

Open fires are often not permitted in the backcountry, especially near lakes, in high-use areas, and during dry times when the Forest Service may issue a fire ban. Backpacking stoves are the prescribed method for cooking in the Tahoe region.

Wildlife, and black bears in particular (see page 20), learn to associate hikers and backpacks with food. It's up to all of us to protect them from becoming dependent on our supplies. Using a canister to protect your food from being nabbed by a bear is far superior to hanging a bear bag. Odor-proof plastic bags, however, are effective in keeping smaller animals out of your food.

Solid human waste must be buried in a hole at least 6 inches deep and at least 200 feet away from trails and water sources; a trowel is basic backpacking equipment. Paper products should never be buried or burned. Instead, carry out your used paper products in a doubled plastic bag and dispose of them at home.

Following the previous guidelines will increase your chances for a pleasant, safe, and low-impact interaction between humans and nature. Forest regulations can change over time, however, so contact the appropriate forest ranger station to check for updates before you enter the backcountry.

Tips on Enjoying Hiking Tahoe

You made the first important decision affecting the successful outcome of your hike by reading this guidebook. Be sure to study the introductory information: The advice here was gained from hiking and climbing in many environments and generally holds true across all of them. The hikes in this guide traverse terrain spanning more than 5,120 feet in elevation while exploring ridges, rivers, lakes, and geological and historical sights.

Prepare for your hike by leaving detailed trip information with an emergency contact and gathering information about the hike from the appropriate agency listed in Appendix A (page 287) or in the "Contacts" listings. Use the overview map on the inside front cover, along with the regional maps at the beginning of each chapter, to determine the locations of alternative hikes, and make sure they match your abilities.

These hikes are rated as *easy, moderate,* or *strenuous.* These ratings—using a five-star system—are completely subjective evaluations based on somewhat objective criteria. You should get some satisfaction, however, in knowing that these hikes were rated by someone with no more than average abilities who arrived from sea level without acclimatization to the majority of the hikes.

EASY HIKES This is Lake Tahoe. It has mountains all around it. Where are you going to find something easy to hike around here? The criteria, hard as they are to find, are simply that the trail be groomed, nearly level, and shorter than 2 miles. The **Tahoe Meadows Interpretive Trail** (page 35) is an easy hike. Add another star to it, and the rating means a longer, graded trail where you may break a momentary sweat. **Lake Margaret** (page 118) seems to fit this description.

MODERATE HIKES Three stars means you'll be hiking more than 5 miles with some ups and downs along the way. If you're a nonsmoker in average physical condition, these hikes will seem easy, but they're a bit more involved and may take more time. Bump the action up by one star, and you enter the "challenging" zone. This could mean more navigational work, a longer trail, steeper inclines, higher elevations, or any combination of those things.

STRENUOUS HIKES Five stars will be everything you imagined. Count on some sustained or steep inclines as well as rocky, long, or missing trails. **Pyramid Peak** (page 147) is short but vertical. It's strenuous. So is **McConnell Lake Loop** (page 206), which is long, rocky, and vertical. See? Incredibly subjective.

Lake Tahoe and the surrounding Sierra Nevada mountains are special in more ways than their rugged beauty. Follow the various permit processes to the letter, and you won't have to retrace your steps prematurely or in the company of a ranger. Having hiked all over the country, I find it satisfying to see well-maintained trails resulting from the fees I've paid. Even the day-hike permits, being free, benefit hikers. First, they let potential rescuers know who went where and when. Second, that same information actually helps the US Forest Service determine its priorities for trail and facility improvements and maintenance.

The signage that the Forest Service uses to identify roads in its domain is fairly simple. And because Lake Tahoe is surrounded by three national forests and borders three wilderness areas, most hikers are very familiar with them. As a reminder, however, the following information can help in navigating to the trailhead:

Main forest roads, such as the road to Wrights Lake (Wrights Lake Road), are noted by a small, square, brown-and-white sign with a numerical Forest Road designation—in the case of Wrights Lake Road, **FR 4,** or simply the number 4 or 04—within the white-bordered square on the brown background.

Signage for **secondary forest roads** is distinct and more descriptive. The sign itself, still Forest Service brown, is a slender, vertically oriented rectangle. For example, one of the secondary forest road signs at the Wrights Lake Visitor Center is labeled **12N23**.

Tertiary forest roads are seen less frequently in this area because they are normally useful only in actively logged areas. None were used in this book to navigate to trailheads.

There are so many locations in the "Tahoe vicinity" that are worth hiking to and writing about that I had to limit my range to a strictly defined area. By drawing a line consistently 25 miles from Lake Tahoe's shore, I defined the area on which to focus my attention. I then divided the resulting amoeba-shaped region into three sections by doing some border-flipping. Mirroring the California–Nevada border yielded three nearly equal areas, placing hikes to the east, west, or south of the lake.

Trail Etiquette

Always treat trails, wildlife, and fellow hikers with respect. Here are some reminders.

★ **PLAN AHEAD IN ORDER TO BE SELF-SUFFICIENT AT ALL TIMES.** For example, carry necessary supplies for changes in weather or other conditions. A well-planned trip brings satisfaction to you and to others.

★ **HIKE ON OPEN TRAILS ONLY.**

★ **RESPECT TRAIL AND ROAD CLOSURES** (check if unsure), avoid possibly trespassing on private land, and obtain all permits and authorization as required. Leave gates as you found them or as marked.

★ **BE COURTEOUS TO OTHER HIKERS,** bikers, equestrians, and others you encounter on the trails.

★ **NEVER SPOOK WILD ANIMALS OR PETS.** An unannounced approach, a sudden movement, or a loud noise startles most critters, and a surprised animal can be dangerous to you, to others, and to itself. Give animals plenty of space.

★ **OBSERVE ANY "YIELD" SIGNS** you encounter. Typically they advise hikers to yield to horses, and bikers to yield to both horses and hikers. Observing common courtesy on hills, hikers and bikers yield to any uphill traffic. When encountering mounted riders or horse-packers, hikers can courteously step off the trail, on the downhill side if possible. Speak to the rider before he or she reaches you, and don't dart behind a tree. (You're less spooky if the horse can see and hear you.) Don't pet horses unless you're invited to do so.

★ **STAY ON THE EXISTING TRAIL,** and don't blaze any new trails.

★ **PACK OUT WHAT YOU PACK IN.** No one wants to see the trash some-one else has left behind. That includes anything your pet may deposit on the trail, so come prepared with a few plastic bags.

SHALLOW MAUD LAKE *(see Hike 28, Lake Lois and Lake Schmidell, page 197)*

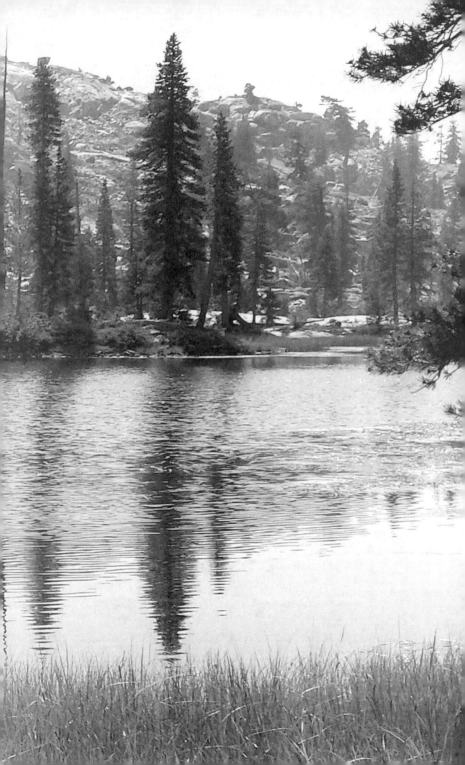

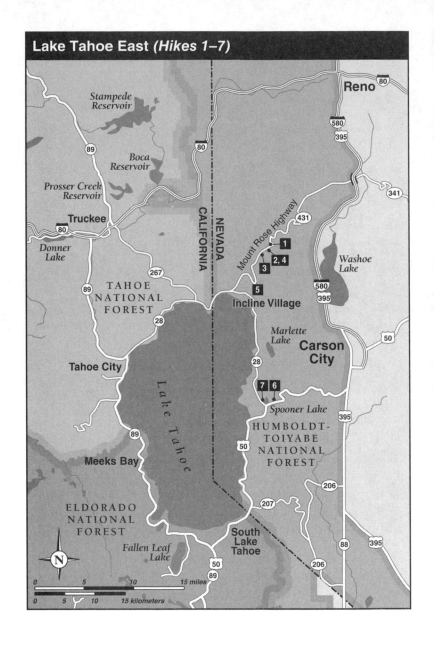

Lake Tahoe East *(Hikes 1–7)*

Reno

Stampede
Reservoir

Boca
Reservoir

Prosser Creek
Reservoir

Truckee

Donner
Lake

CALIFORNIA

NEVADA

Mount Rose Highway

1

2, 4

3

Washoe
Lake

5

Incline Village

TAHOE
NATIONAL
FOREST

Tahoe City

Marlette
Lake

Carson
City

Lake Tahoe

7 **6**

Spooner Lake

HUMBOLDT-
TOIYABE
NATIONAL
FOREST

Meeks Bay

ELDORADO
NATIONAL
FOREST

Fallen Leaf
Lake

South Lake
Tahoe

N

0   5   10   15 miles
0   5   10   15 kilometers

Lake Tahoe East

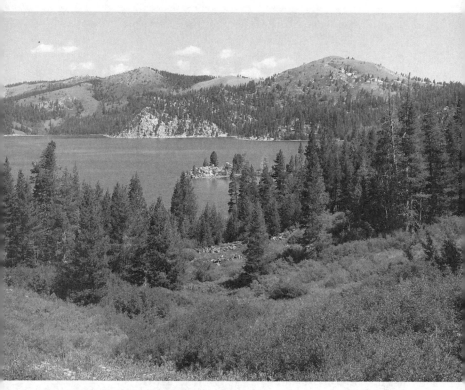

MARLETTE LAKE FROM THE FOOTBRIDGE *(see Hike 6, page 56)*

Mount Rose

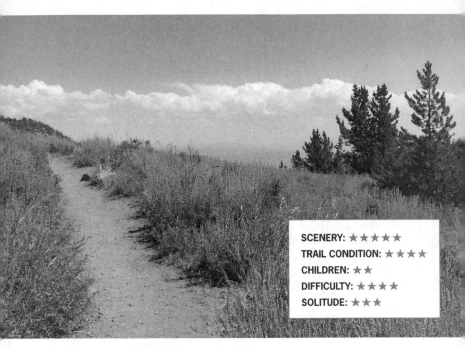

SCENERY: ★★★★★
TRAIL CONDITION: ★★★★
CHILDREN: ★★
DIFFICULTY: ★★★★
SOLITUDE: ★★★

MIDWAY EN ROUTE TO MOUNT ROSE'S SUMMIT

GPS TRAILHEAD COORDINATES: N39° 18.768′ W119° 53.849′

DISTANCE & CONFIGURATION: 10.2-mile out-and-back

HIKING TIME: 5–7 hours

OUTSTANDING FEATURES: Pleasant trail through pine forest, plus a waterfall beneath Mount Houghton. A well-defined trail leads to the summit for a 360-degree view all the way from Stampede Reservoir in the west to the Carson Range in the east, with Lake Tahoe laid out for 22 blue miles below you to the south.

ELEVATION: 8,904′ at trailhead

ACCESS: Year-round

MAPS: *Lake Tahoe Basin* (Trails Illustrated 803)

FACILITIES: Pit toilet

COMMENTS: Carry water.

CONTACT: Humboldt-Toiyabe National Forest, Carson Ranger District, 775-882-2766, www.fs.usda.gov/htnf

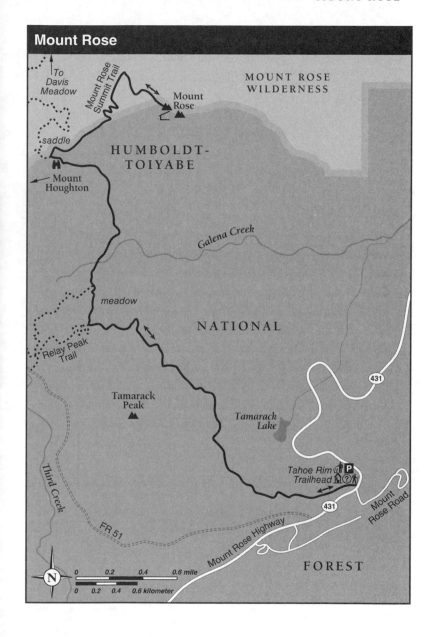

Mount Rose

To Davis Meadow

Mount Rose Summit Trail

MOUNT ROSE WILDERNESS

Mount Rose

saddle

HUMBOLDT-TOIYABE

Mount Houghton

Galena Creek

meadow

NATIONAL

Relay Peak Trail

Tamarack Peak

Tamarack Lake

431

Tahoe Rim Trailhead

Third Creek

FR 51

431

Mount Rose Highway

Mount Rose Road

FOREST

N

| 0 | 0.2 | 0.4 | 0.6 mile |

| 0 | 0.2 | 0.4 | 0.6 kilometer |

Overview

This trail is straightforward and pleasant to walk the entire way. You'll use a ridge at the foot of Mount Houghton to gain 200 feet in the first 0.5 mile before crossing that ridge to traverse for the next 2 miles with no elevation gain. You'll have great views of Lake Tahoe initially before your destination begins to dominate the vista. The final 2.5 miles to the summit are interrupted only by a few switchbacks up the more than 1,700 feet to the top of this old volcano.

Route Details

No one is certain about the origin of Mount Rose's name—even whether it came from a man or a woman. But we do know that Church Peak, the twin summit on this ridge, honors Dr. James Church of the University of Nevada, who established the first high-altitude meteorological observatory here and developed the modern science of snow survey, which is used today. At 10,776 feet, Mount Rose is the highest point around Lake Tahoe's Nevada side.

Walk past the pit toilets to the trailhead, which is situated immediately behind them at the kiosk. Less than 100 feet past the trailhead is the hikers-only trailhead for the Tahoe Rim Trail, which leads to the Mount Rose Summit Trail. The Tahoe Rim Trail

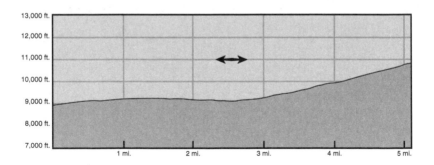

Association supplies trail maps at the kiosk, where hikers can also read up on preferred wilderness practices.

Head uphill with a sharp turn at the kiosk, and immediately take in the views to the south and west, where Lake Tahoe comes into view. In exactly 0.5 mile, the trail will level out. Conveniently enough, you'll find a tight formation of boulders shaded by pine, perfect for putting on the sunscreen that you forgot to apply in the parking lot. The broad, sandy, well-marked trail stays level, or nearly so, meandering across a lightly treed, south-facing slope for the next 2 miles as you traverse to the northwest of Tamarack Lake. You may cross a couple of runoff streams as you get sneak peeks of Mount Rose at about 1.25 miles along, and in another 0.5 mile, you have a clear view of your destination as you walk along a steep slope.

Just before the trail's 2.5-mile midpoint, the Tahoe Rim Trail veers to the west toward Relay Peak. At the next fork in the trail, momentarily leave your route on the path to your left, which leads over to a rocky cascade and an opportunity to refill your water. Don't miss this cool photo opportunity. Continue on your route to the right and cross the stream on boulders placed there for you, then on through this marshy area along the rock-and-gravel causeway. The trail continues north beneath a power line, next to a large meadow with beautiful views down the canyon to the east. Just after you crash through the willows and lupine at the next stream, you'll pass another junction where the Tahoe Rim Trail diverges from our route and heads to Relay Peak.

From this intersection, climb across one of Mount Houghton's eastern flanks, and then begin ascending the crease between it and Mount Rose. Climb these tree-covered slopes, then cross to the north side of the ravine and resume hiking up the rock-filled ditch to a saddle 400 feet above. Just as you reach the saddle, you will encounter the boundary sign for the Mount Rose Wilderness. At the saddle, continue to walk around it 150 feet to the west to reach the end of a ridge, which you will mount and hike to the northeast. Ignore the trail junction to Thomas Creek Trailhead—this is a segment of the Mount Rose Trail heading to Davis Meadow.

Turn uphill to the right. Your destination lies 1 mile ahead. The dirt-and-rock trail becomes somewhat scrabbly as it ascends the prominent ridge rather directly. After reaching the first switchback in 0.5 mile, you may enjoy the chance to take in the scenery (along with some extra oxygen). The switchbacks will lead you to a traverse of the northwest slope, where you will turn southeast on the lower portion of the summit ridge. Three final switchbacks through the rocks carry you up to the ridge and a simple 250-foot walk to the summit.

The shelters here protect you somewhat from the wind. The thousands of California tortoiseshell butterflies are apparently unaffected by these gusts. There are two perches of similar height here; both offer spectacular vistas of Boca, Stampede, and Prosser Reservoirs to the northwest, Mount Houghton and Relay Peak to the southwest, and Washoe Lake to the east.

Directions

From Truckee, take I-80 east 2.5 miles to CA 267/CA 89, Exit 188B, toward Lake Tahoe. Drive 11.6 miles and turn left on CA 28. Drive 4.6 miles on CA 28 before turning left onto Mount Rose Highway/NV 431. Drive 8.2 miles uphill to Mount Rose Road, where a large parking lot is on the left.

From I-80 in Reno, drive 10 miles south on US 395 to Mount Rose Highway/NV 431, and then drive 16 miles east to the summit parking lot.

Pit toilets and trash receptacles are available at the top of this year-round pass.

2 # Tahoe Meadows Interpretive Trail

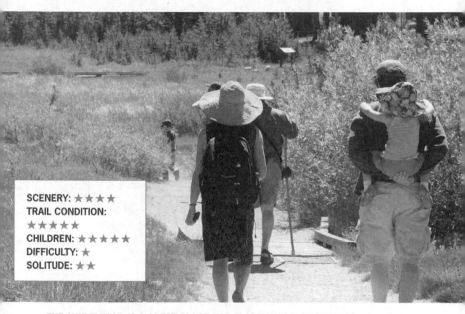

THE SUNLIT TRAIL IS A GREAT PLACE FOR FLOPPY-HAT FASHION. Photo: Stacy Laughlin

SCENERY: ★ ★ ★ ★
TRAIL CONDITION:
★ ★ ★ ★ ★
CHILDREN: ★ ★ ★ ★ ★
DIFFICULTY: ★
SOLITUDE: ★ ★

GPS TRAILHEAD COORDINATES: N39° 18.439′ W119° 54.433′

DISTANCE & CONFIGURATION: 1.4-mile loop

HIKING TIME: 30–60 minutes

OUTSTANDING FEATURES: This wonderfully situated interpretive trail overlooks Tahoe Meadows. Broad trail on gentle terrain has a great overlook and excellent displays describing the flora, fauna, and natural history of the meadows.

ELEVATION: 8,691′ at trailhead

ACCESS: Depends on snow

MAPS: *Tahoe Rim Trail* (Tom Harrison Maps)

FACILITIES: Pit toilet

COMMENTS: This accessible trail—the only one in this book—traverses around and overlooks a magnificent subalpine meadow.

CONTACT: Humboldt-Toiyabe National Forest, Carson Ranger District, 775-882-2766, www.fs.usda.gov/htnf

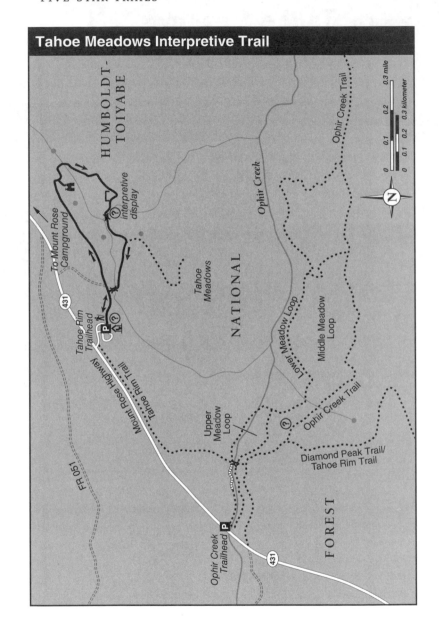

Tahoe Meadows Interpretive Trail

Overview

The Tahoe Meadows Interpretive Loop packs a lot of nature into 1.4 miles. This well-engineered trail provides hikers of all ages and abilities access to a prototypal meadow ecosystem. All sizes of wild-life abound in this subalpine meadow adorned with streams, ringed by trees, and lush with flowers. A viewing platform overlooks this expansive terrain. Bring your binoculars.

Route Details

Your journey along the interpretive trail begins at the kiosk next to the trees, directly east of the pit toilets. Head east on the trail as it leaves the shade, and bear right onto the path ahead. You actually follow the Tahoe Rim Trail as it leads to Mount Rose Campground. This grass-surrounded track features several bridges that enable wheel-chair access around the loop. The first is just about 400 feet along and spans a tiny stream running out of the copse of trees 50 feet to the north. The broad, sandy trail passes the meadow that sprouts lodgepole pines as well as willows.

Just ahead is a junction featuring an interpretive display—an overview of the species routinely spotted here. Wildflowers vary throughout the season, as do migrating birds. This meadow is a

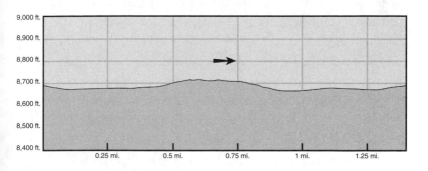

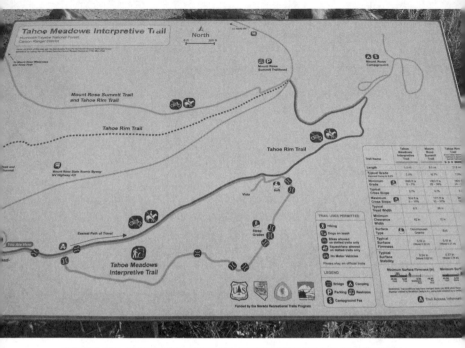

SIGNAGE AND INTERPRETIVE DISPLAYS ARE INFORMATIVE AND EDUCATIONAL.

favorite area for birders to set up their own perches for observing. The easiest direction on this loop leads straight ahead, past the point where the loop rejoins this path. The boulders to the left of the junction are a good habitat for the Belding's ground squirrels that are constantly on the lookout for the red-tailed hawks cruising overhead.

The trail signage points out the trail width, composition, cross-slope, and grade—important information for wheelchair hikers. The next slight grade leads across another small rivulet before the track reveals its asphalt past. The trail gains just enough elevation to enable hikers to look down into the meadow to the right. The former roadbed is outlined by pussypaws, paintbrush, and sage and is pleasantly shaded by some magnificent lodgepole pines. A spring keeps the sand ahead somewhat damp, but that also makes it firmer underfoot.

As Mount Rose comes into view, your track bears right and leaves the Tahoe Rim Trail. A hundred feet hence is an engineered spur trail leading to a vista point. Next to this overlook is a double lodgepole surrounded on three sides by meadow and facing the tree-spotted knoll to the southwest. Return to the loop and cross two bridges spanning the creek, where you can spot small brook trout. The return leg heads south along the meadow's margin, staying just inside the trees at the foot of Slide Mountain. Bridges span each streamlet as you walk beneath the pines. After pausing at one restful bench, the trail jogs west between two small knolls.

The meadow here is ringed with broad, sandy slopes, which, like the meadow itself, are a result of glacial action in the not-too-distant past. Follow the path under Western white pine and some mature hemlocks as you stay under tree cover for the next 150 yards. Looking into the meadow from the south toward its wet core allows patient observers to see raccoon and coyotes and maybe a black bear. Cross the causeway, and a final left returns you to the trailhead.

Directions

Leave Incline Village on Mount Rose Highway/NV 431 and drive 7.4 miles to the Tahoe Meadows Trailhead parking lot, on the east side of the road. Vault toilets are available, but water and trash service are not. The Tahoe Rim Trail is marked by a kiosk to the west of the pit toilets. You can pick up a trail map here.

The trailhead for the Interpretive Loop is across the parking lot, east of the pit toilets. It's marked by an informational kiosk and a map display describing the trail.

Tahoe Meadows Trails

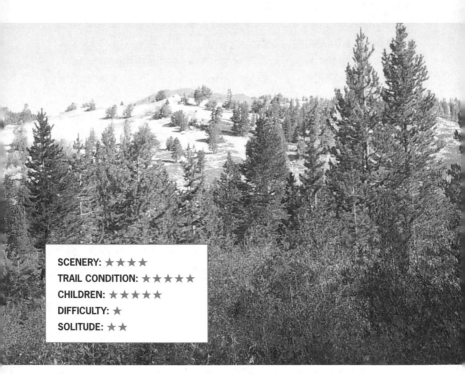

SCENERY: ★ ★ ★ ★
TRAIL CONDITION: ★ ★ ★ ★ ★
CHILDREN: ★ ★ ★ ★ ★
DIFFICULTY: ★
SOLITUDE: ★ ★

LOWER MEADOW LOOP OFFERS VIEWS EAST FROM ABOVE THE MEADOW'S EDGE.

GPS TRAILHEAD COORDINATES: N39° 18.443′ W119° 54.484′

DISTANCE & CONFIGURATION: 1.5–4.5-mile loops

HIKING TIME: 2–3 hours

OUTSTANDING FEATURES: Subalpine meadow teeming with flowers and wildlife; three trails along pristine stream to match family hiker levels.

ELEVATION: 8,538′ at trailhead

ACCESS: Year-round

MAPS: *Tahoe Rim Trail* (Tom Harrison Maps)

FACILITIES: Pit toilet

CONTACT: Humboldt-Toiyabe National Forest, Carson Ranger District, 775-882-2766, www.fs.usda.gov/htnf

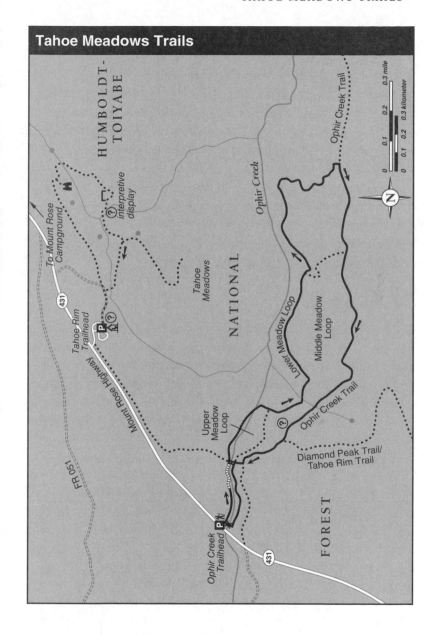

Tahoe Meadows Trails

HUMBOLDT-
TOIYABE

NATIONAL

FOREST

Tahoe Meadows

Ophir Creek

Ophir Creek Trail

Lower Meadow Loop

Middle Meadow Loop

Upper Meadow Loop

Ophir Creek Trail

Diamond Peak Trail/
Tahoe Rim Trail

To Mount Rose
Campground

interpretive
display

Mount Rose Highway

Tahoe Rim Trailhead

FR 051

Ophir Creek Trailhead

431

431

0.3 mile
0.1   0.2
0   0.1   0.2   0.3 kilometer

N

Overview

The paths that meander around Tahoe Meadows are covered with footprints and signs of mammals, the air is filled with songbirds and raptors, and the ground is alive with masses of wildflowers and trees. This hike has no particular destination, and it's not going to get you anywhere other than familiar with nature. A natural-history field guide would be a welcome companion on this walk, because you'll have a chance to use it often.

You can hike along Ophir Creek as it winds through the larger Tahoe Meadows. A combination of natural surfaces and composition boardwalk allows hikers to observe this natural area without disturbing the fragile soils and plants. Hikers are strongly encouraged to keep their pets under control in this sensitive area.

Route Details

Tahoe Meadows offers three trails to explore. If you parked along Mount Rose Highway, take the stairs down the bank to the trails. If you parked in the lot up the hill, embark from the informational kiosk at the Tahoe Rim Trail Trailhead near Mount Rose Highway just 200 feet west of the pit toilets. As you walk along, watch for red-tailed hawks soaring above the meadow, usually on their way to a higher perch but sometimes on a mission, talons poised for lunch. The sand-and-gravel trail is bound by a log fence on the left and Mount Rose

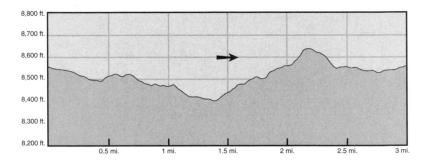

Highway on the right. The path veers left, angling across the meadow, toward the footbridge at Ophir Creek.

Hikers can observe the meadow from two viewpoints: as they walk along the creek within the meadow and looking in on it from the treed margins of this open space. To preserve the meadow's plant life and control streamside soil erosion, dedicated conservationists and Tahoe Rim Trail Association volunteers have installed bridges and built causeways and boardwalks. The trails in the meadow are connected to one another but do not have to be followed in any order. However, this is a fragile ecosystem with established trails. Wherever you walk, strictly observe the paths (including controlling your pets and picking up after them).

The excellent signage displays a map with all three trails. The Upper Meadow Loop begins close to the stairs at the trailhead marker reading WEST TAHOE MEADOWS LOOP TRAILS. This loop stays close to Ophir Creek, where there's plenty of activity among the streamside grasses and submerged rocks. All three loops share the tread in the area from the footbridge to the stairs.

The Middle Meadow Loop mirrors the longer Lower Meadow Loop, but it stops about 0.3 mile earlier, so it's slightly shorter at 2.3 miles. Both climb more into the forest to the south of the meadows. The Lower Meadow Loop is 3 miles around, and that is the loop that this hike follows. But any of these is spectacular regardless of what direction it's hiked. First, the Upper Meadow Loop, which is a great trail for wobbly little-hiker legs.

Starting at the trailhead, follow the trail east along the north side of the creek. A boardwalk protects the fragile zone next to this stream to prevent bank cave-ins, erosion, and loss of vegetation due to trampling. Halfway along this slope into the meadow, you'll find a nice footbridge over the Ophir. This is a great spot to linger, as small trout seem to flash by here as if on cue. Still heading east on engineered tread, corn lilies, buttercups, and paintbrush add color and fragrance to the banks of this briskly bubbling creek.

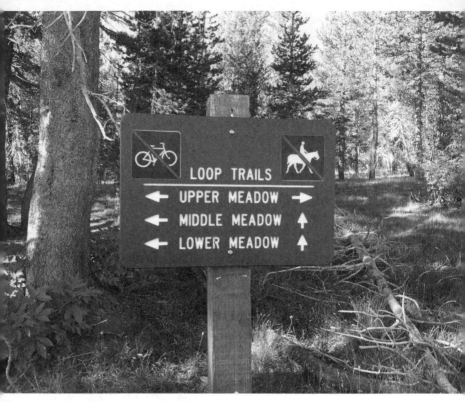

THREE CONNECTED LOOP TRAILS OFFER A HIKE SURE TO BE ENJOYED BY HIKERS OF EVERY AGE.

After 0.2 mile, the Lower Meadow Loop Trail continues ahead and the Upper Meadow Trail turns right, now heading west, back to the trailhead. If you take this alternate return, some quick elevation gain allows you to see into the meadow and over your shoulder as you walk to the northwest. The trail stays just inside the trees except for a sandy area just before the creek. Rejoin the creek at the footbridge and head west on the shaded south bank until you reach the trailhead in 0.2 mile.

You will certainly gain different perspectives by venturing along the 3-mile-long Lower Meadow Loop Trail. Continue past the Upper

Meadow Loop return, heading south and then east into this sloping meadow. The trail stays inside the trees as your route skirts a lightly treed area about 100 yards south of the creek. After 0.6 mile, you will pass the return leg for the Middle Meadow Loop. About 50 feet later, your trail requires crossing a rocky ravine as you continue east. The boulder-lined trail meanders along the forest's margin, allowing you to gaze down on Ophir Creek.

This loop's return leg starts with a curvy 90-degree course change to the south. A quarter of a mile and 75 feet of vertical gain later, you will intersect the Ophir Creek Trail, which is your route west, back to the trailhead. Now traveling with the hill on your right, enjoy the shaded trail under a canopy of lodgepole and Western white pines.

The meadow flowers disappear, but the forest is no less brightly colored, thanks to the brilliant red snow plants. Graze the small meadow to your left and step over its small runoff stream. In just 200 yards, watch for an information kiosk alongside the trail; 100 yards past the kiosk, you'll reach the intersection with the Tahoe Rim Trail section that leads to Diamond Peak to the south. To get back to the bridge at Ophir Creek, follow your trail straight ahead, northwest, about 0.25 mile, and then hook a sharp right at the junction that leads you over to the bridge.

Directions

Leave Incline Village on Mount Rose Highway/NV 431 and drive 6.7 miles to the West Tahoe Meadows Loop Trails trailhead parking area, which is anywhere along the east side of the road. Two sets of stairs lead down to the trails. The stairs farthest west are closest to the trailhead.

Additional parking is available in the lot on the east side of Mount Rose Highway at the Tahoe Meadows Interpretive Trail, which is 0.7 mile up the hill toward Mount Rose. A connector trail will lead you to the Tahoe Meadows trails.

Diamond Peak

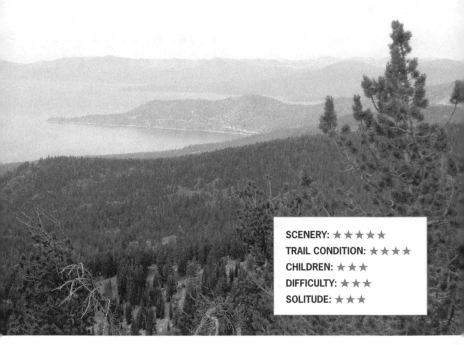

SCENERY: ★ ★ ★ ★ ★
TRAIL CONDITION: ★ ★ ★ ★
CHILDREN: ★ ★ ★
DIFFICULTY: ★ ★ ★
SOLITUDE: ★ ★ ★

CRYSTAL AND AGATE BAYS FROM THE TAHOE RIM TRAIL AT DIAMOND PEAK

GPS TRAILHEAD COORDINATES: N39° 18.442′ W119° 54.484′

DISTANCE & CONFIGURATION: 11-mile out-and-back

HIKING TIME: 6 hours

OUTSTANDING FEATURES: This hike starts in a flower-filled meadow and just gets better. It features some incredible vistas of Lake Tahoe from secluded outcrops, and the trail, despite short ups and downs, is sandy, level, and pleasantly shaded by firs and pines.

ELEVATION: 8,563′ at trailhead

ACCESS: Depends on snow

MAPS: *Tahoe Rim Trail* (Tom Harrison Maps)

FACILITIES: Toilet

CONTACT: Humboldt-Toiyabe National Forest, Carson Ranger District, 775-882-2766, www.fs.usda.gov/htnf

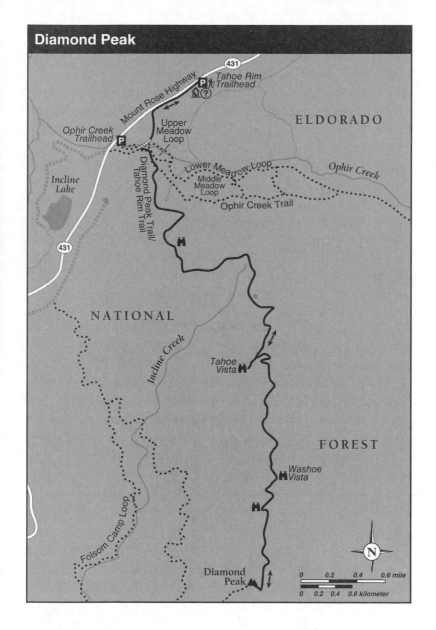

Diamond Peak

431

Mount Rose Highway

Tahoe Rim Trailhead

P

ELDORADO

Ophir Creek Trailhead

P

Upper Meadow Loop

Lower Meadow Loop

Ophir Creek

Incline Lake

Diamond Peak Trail/ Tahoe Rim Trail

Middle Meadow Loop

Ophir Creek Trail

431

NATIONAL

Incline Creek

Tahoe Vista

FOREST

Washoe Vista

Folsom Camp Loop

Diamond Peak

N

0   0.2   0.4   0.6 mile

0   0.2   0.4   0.6 kilometer

Overview

Tahoe Meadows is a wonderful trailhead—one of the most pleasant around the lake—from which to embark on a day hike. The route to Diamond Peak is mostly level, gaining the ridge in about 300 feet and then generally following it south through forests of Western white pine, lodgepole pine, red fir, and Jeffrey pine. The high point of the hike is slightly above 8,800 feet, while the destination is at 8,540 feet (and has a chairlift terminus attached to it). For the most solitude, avoid even-numbered days, when mountain bikes have access to this excellent trail.

Route Details

Embark from the information kiosk for the Tahoe Rim Trail (TRT) at the northwest corner of the trailhead parking lot. The obvious trail to the southwest parallels Mount Rose Highway and skirts the meadow for 0.4 mile. As you approach Ophir Creek, causeways assist your trek across the wet ground and around the fragile plants. Cross the footbridge and follow signs for the TRT.

Shortly after you enter the trees, a couple of rapid left–right turns at the signed intersections will point you southeast on the TRT. The next junction to watch for is 1,000 feet ahead, where the Ophir Creek Trail veers left and you and the TRT, bound for Tunnel Creek Road, slide right.

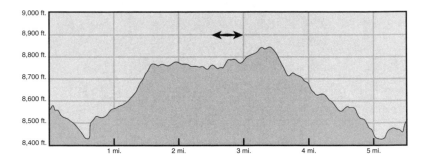

The sandy trail heads south under lodgepole cover 0.3 mile, after which it heads east on the first of two long switchbacks that lead to a good vista of Lake Tahoe. Additional vistas are more frequent as the trees thin out and the boulders replace them. Walk south until the trail turns across the spur of the ridge, tracks east about 0.5 mile, and then resumes its southerly course.

After nearly 3 miles, you can find a reliable water source at the spring just above the trail. Contour south another 0.5 mile to a small clearing. There, an obvious social trail leads 400 feet southwest to an outcrop with a perch at about 8,830 feet affording a spectacular view over Lake Tahoe. Crystal Bay stretches in front of you, with Agate Bay in the background. Crystal Bay was named not for its gemlike waters but for George Crystal, who staked the first claim on timber here in the 1860s. This is an excellent spot for a snack or lunch break.

Return to the trail and continue in and out of a ravine as you descend slightly from the high point of 8,830 feet. Contour in and out of the canyon among boulders on a sandy trail. Penstemon, pinemat manzanita, buckwheat, and pussypaws are the only colorful additions on this boulder-ridden slope. Descend into a broad, flat saddle ringed by lodgepole pine, Western white pine, and red fir trees. Hidden from the Tahoe side, vistas into the Washoe Valley and shallow Washoe Lake appear to the east as you descend the sandy trail.

From the next brief vista on the Tahoe side, you can spot the trip's destination, highlighted by the chairlift terminus. Descend to another small, almost circular, saddle, where you will begin to contour along the eastern side of Diamond Peak. A faint trail heads southwest up through the trees (just before they completely peter out) to the peak. Or you can round the curve 400 feet farther south and then, just before entering the saddle, turn uphill on the sandy slope to your destination.

The return to the trailhead is easier, and any missed pictures are still there.

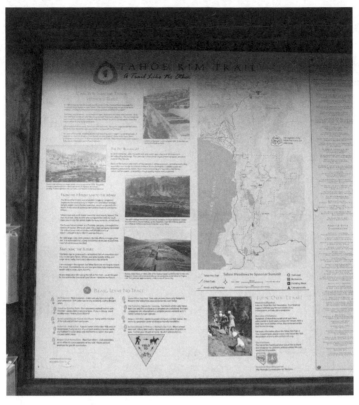

INFORMATIVE KIOSKS AT TRAILHEADS AROUND THE LAKE ARE MAINTAINED BY TAHOE RIM TRAIL ASSOCIATION VOLUNTEERS.

Directions

Leave Incline Village on Mount Rose Highway/NV 431 and drive 7.4 miles to the Tahoe Meadows Trailhead parking lot, on the east side of the road. Pit toilets are available, but water and garbage service are not. This is about 0.75 mile past the stairs that lead more directly to the trail, but this way you have a pretty meadow to walk in and you can leave your car in the worry-free TRT trailhead parking lot. If the lot is full, park on the south side of the highway, 0.75 mile back toward the lake.

5

Folsom Camp Loop

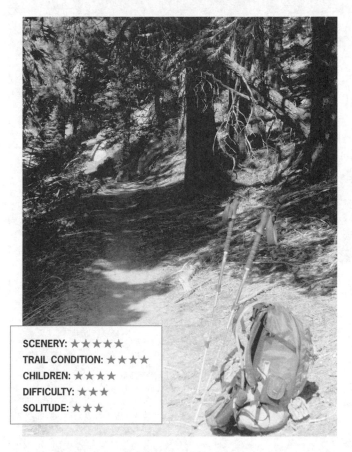

SCENERY: ★ ★ ★ ★ ★
TRAIL CONDITION: ★ ★ ★ ★
CHILDREN: ★ ★ ★ ★
DIFFICULTY: ★ ★
SOLITUDE: ★ ★ ★

GPS TRAILHEAD COORDINATES: N39° 15.219´ W119° 55.393´

DISTANCE & CONFIGURATION: 6.2-mile loop

HIKING TIME: 3–4 hours

OUTSTANDING FEATURES: Historic flume; Tahoe vistas; wildflower-filled meadows

ELEVATION: 6,829´ at trailhead

ACCESS: Year-round

MAPS: *Lake Tahoe Basin* (Trails Illustrated 803)

FACILITIES: None

CONTACT: Humboldt-Toiyabe National Forest, Carson Ranger District, 775-882-2766,
www.fs.usda.gov/htnf

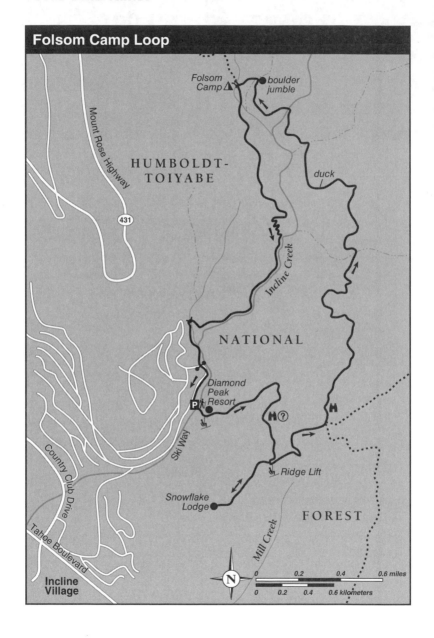

Folsom Camp Loop

Folsom Camp △ ● boulder jumble

HUMBOLDT-TOIYABE

Mount Rose Highway

431

duck

Incline Creek

NATIONAL

Diamond Peak Resort

P

Ski Way

Snowflake Lodge

Ridge Lift

Country Club Drive

Tahoe Boulevard

Incline Village

Mill Creek

FOREST

N

| 0 | 0.2 | 0.4 | 0.6 miles |
| 0 | 0.2 | 0.4 | 0.6 kilometers |

Overview

This loop is easy enough because the length of the trail runs along a historic flume that formerly delivered cordwood and timber to the Washoe Valley. The route is described in the way I initially hiked it, but it might be even easier to hike in reverse. You'll encounter a few steep spots along the described route, but they're not long, and the total elevation gain is 800 feet over 1.3 miles, or 1.75 miles if done in reverse. The middle 3 miles are essentially flat and shaded.

Route Details

Look for the unofficial trailhead near the stairs to the children's ski school, right in front of the lodge at Diamond Peak Resort. Circle past the Crystal Express chairlift and begin gaining elevation along the service road as it winds up to the northeast across moist meadows. Moments after coming abreast of another lift, the road will begin to swing around in the opposite direction, crossing a ski run and a small ridge where you'll have an excellent vista of Lake Tahoe along with an informational display.

When you reach the loading station for Ridge Lift, you can regain your normal breathing pattern while deciding on a short side trip over to Snowflake Lodge, where you have some excellent views

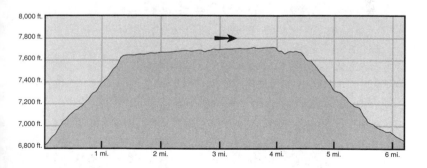

over the lake. To get there, walk 0.35 mile southwest, past a chairlift and a maintenance garage. This is an excellent destination in and of itself, where you can see the Carolina-blue waters of Crystal Bay, as well as Agate Bay (past Stateline Lookout). If this scratches your ooh-and-ahh itch, head back down and call it a great day.

The described hike heads in the opposite direction, northeast about 0.4 mile, and the views will be just as stunning. Pass Luggi's Run, named for Diamond Peak founder Luggi Foegger, as the road meanders under the Ridge Lift. Head to the lift's off-loading area and continue steeply uphill 100 feet. There, the trail on the left will become obvious just as you reach it because the hill flattens for a brief few feet.

Turn north on this level path that maintains the 7,650-foot contour for about the next 3 miles. Take advantage of the photo opportunities over the next few hundred feet, before the Jeffrey pines thicken around you. The views out to the lake are excellent. As you come to a quartet of standing snags, you'll pass beneath the Crystal Express yet again. As you look around, don't forget to look down—for remnants of the original flumeworks, constructed to supply the mines and homes of the Comstock Lode and Virginia City with timber and cordwood. At least 300 cords a day were sent from the slopes of Mill Creek, first up the Incline Railway and then by V-shaped flume through the Virginia and Gold Hill water tunnel.

Cross the last four ski runs of Diamond Peak and amble among the Jeffrey pines with their pungent butterscotch aroma. Notice the sap-laden cones that crown red firs; they actually gleam in the sunlight. As you cross runoff streams, you'll see aspens decorated with carvings of past romances and birthdays alongside willows and ferns, all punctuated by the red berries of mountain ash.

Cross a few runoff streams that augmented the old flume, and then hike west around a ridge spur; continue north across a few more runoff crossings employing old flume materials for bridgeworks. The second of these is one branch of the nascent Incline Creek.

Another stream just 0.3 mile hence drops from sight beneath a jumble of hefty boulders—almost uniformly 2 meters in diameter—just as it reaches the trail. Your trail turns south and crosses another branch of Incline Creek, soon crossing an open area that looks broad and flat enough for a large campsite. In fact, this was Folsom Camp, named for the lumberman Gilman Folsom, who, in partnership with Sam Marlette, supplied some 40,000 cords of wood per year and employed more than 400 Chinese lumbermen in the enterprise.

Continue past Folsom Camp, and cross Incline Creek once again. The trail leading to the northwest continues uphill to Tahoe Meadows. Soon turn south and meander through the lodgepole and fir forest on a sandy trail. The path widens somewhat and follows Incline Creek. As it descends to the condominium complex near the resort, watch for increasing signs of beaver activity along the creek. A footbridge will ease your last crossing, but the creek will keep you company as you turn straight south again after you bump into the condos. A locked chain across the trail is the end of this ride. Step over and walk down the road 0.2 mile to the upper lot.

Directions

Head east from Incline Village on Tahoe Boulevard 2 miles. Turn left onto Country Club Drive. In 0.1 mile, turn right onto Ski Way and drive 1.3 miles to the upper lot at Diamond Peak Resort, where hikers are allowed to park in the summer. The trailhead is in front of the new lodge, below you and to the left.

6 # Marlette Lake

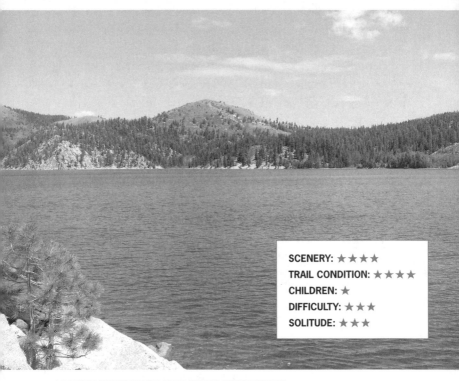

LOOKING NORTH FROM MARLETTE'S SOUTH SHORE.

GPS TRAILHEAD COORDINATES: N39° 06.278′ W119° 53.817′

DISTANCE & CONFIGURATION: 11.6-mile out-and-back

HIKING TIME: 4–6 hours

OUTSTANDING FEATURES: A little bit of history on your way up the gentle grade, with wildlife, wildflowers, aspen groves, and a lakeside trail to amble along

ELEVATION: 7,051′ at trailhead

ACCESS: Year-round; $10 entrance fee April 15–October $15, $7 otherwise

MAPS: *Tahoe Rim Trail* (Tom Harrison Maps)

FACILITIES: Pit toilet

CONTACT: Lake Tahoe Nevada State Park, 775-831-0494, parks.nv.gov/parks /marlette-hobart-backcountry

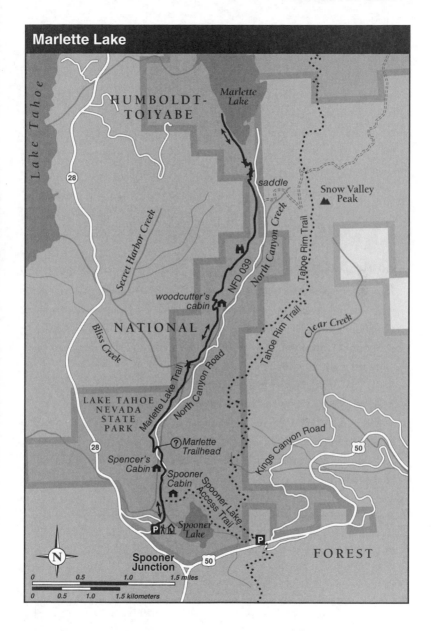

Marlette Lake

Lake Tahoe

HUMBOLDT-
TOIYABE

Marlette
Lake

28

Secret Harbor Creek

saddle

Snow Valley
Peak

North Canyon Creek

NFD 039

Tahoe Rim Trail

woodcutter's
cabin

Bliss Creek

NATIONAL

North Canyon Road

Tahoe Rim Trail

Clear Creek

LAKE TAHOE
NEVADA
STATE
PARK

Marlette Lake Trail

(?) Marlette
Trailhead

28

Kings Canyon Road

50

Spencer's
Cabin

Spooner
Cabin

Spooner Lake
Access Trail

P

FOREST

P

Spooner
Lake

N

Spooner
Junction

50

0   0.5   1.0   1.5 miles
0   0.5   1.0   1.5 kilometers

Overview

Watch for this trail to be one of the first to be clear of snow, rewarding early-season hikers with trailside flowers and spectacular views of two lakes that were once part of the famous flume system that supplied water to Virginia City from the 1870s into the 1900s. Deer, owls, goshawks, Steller's jays, flickers, and chickadees are plentiful on this pleasant and conveniently located hike. Pass Spencer's Cabin on North Canyon Road, which leads to the Marlette Lake Trailhead. While the trail initially gains some elevation, the 1,200-foot climb to the saddle above Marlette Lake is one of the gentlest uphill paths on the east side of the lake. A gentle descent leads to the lake's southern inlet stream.

Route Details

From the trailhead at the Lake Tahoe Nevada State Park parking lot, walk 0.1 mile east to join North Canyon Road. In another 0.2 mile, the Spooner Lake Trail intersects from the right. If you chose to park at Spooner Summit and embark from that trailhead, this is where you will turn right and head north.

In 0.3 mile, you will see Spencer's Cabin on the left. This cabin was formerly used by the caretaker of the ranch owned in the early 1900s by Charlie Fulstone. Now used as a summertime rest stop and as a warming hut for wintertime travelers, it's open to all users and has a working woodburning stove. A Leave No Trace attitude is all that the park asks.

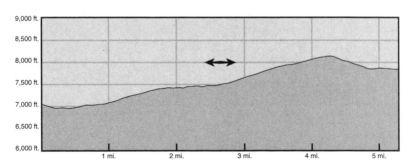

In another 300 paces, you will see an informational kiosk and the formal trailhead for the Marlette Lake Trail. As the sign says, this is a moderate hike, and you will reach your goal in 3.75 miles. At this point, hikers and equestrians head uphill through the trees on the west side of the canyon, while bicyclists continue their climb on the road.

As your path winds uphill, the Jeffrey and lodgepole pines will help keep you shaded and cool on this duff-and-sand trail. Your track is bordered by fragrant lupine and silvery woolly mule's ears. When the trail turns to sand and the canopy opens up above you, you can't help but notice the wind rattling the aspens on the opposite side of the meadow. Your path will cross North Canyon Creek a few times along the way, with the aid of sturdy footbridges.

A good spot to filter water is at the first footbridge, but there are three other decent spots before the lake: 0.5 mile farther on, next to the woodcutter's cabin, or on the other side of the saddle at two or three stream crossings. While this hike is largely shaded, the sun is intense during those times you're exposed. Carry sunscreen and apply it early in this hike. Because the sun reflects off the rock and snow, apply sunscreen to the back of your legs (if you're wearing shorts) and especially to the underside of your chin, ears, and nose.

Your trail switchbacks and points you northeast after you leave the woodcutter's cabin. If you're here early in the day, listen for the sound of flickers hammering at the standing snags in search of yummy grubs. After an hour of hiking, you may begin to interpret the call of the mountain chickadee—the "cheeseburger bird" that flies all around you in aspens or pines. For some excellent views of snowcapped peaks, look back, at about 8,000 feet in elevation, for the vista framed through the trees. If you miss it on the way in, the vista will be framed by the trees and the trail as you return home.

If you're intrepid enough to search for higher vistas, look east for the Tahoe Rim Trail heading up to Snow Valley Peak. Six gentle switchbacks carry you up the 1,000 feet to the peak. You can access that trail just before you reach the saddle above Marlette Lake. The hike continues past the saddle about 300 feet downhill to Marlette Lake's inlet.

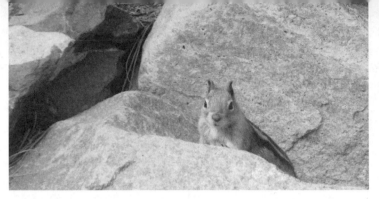

GOLDEN-MANTLED GROUND SQUIRRELS ARE CUTE, BUT THEY'RE PROS AT STEALING FOOD.

Douglas-firs add to the shade on this hillside leading down to Marlette Lake. From your uphill vantage point, you'll have a couple of beautiful views of the lake. You will also see the fish ladders for the trout hatchery at the inlet stream on the lake's south end.

Marlette Lake was held in private hands from its inception as a reservoir for the Hobart-Marlette flume system. For decades it has been a popular trout-fishing destination. While the Lahontin cut-throat trout are no longer favored, brook trout and rainbow trout are spawned and raised in these streams.

From this point at the lake's inlet, you can turn left and walk 1.4 miles along the west edge of the lake to the vistas of Lake Tahoe from the dam and the Flume Trail bike path. Explore either side of the lake on the bike path. Return to the trailhead by retracing your steps.

Directions

From Carson City, drive south on US 395 to US 50 West, then drive 9.8 miles to NV 28 South. Turn right and drive 0.7 mile to Lake Tahoe Nevada State Park. Entrance fees apply here.

From Incline Village, drive 9.3 miles south on NV 28 to Lake Tahoe Nevada State Park, on the east side of the road. If you're starting on the Spooner Lake Trail, continue 0.7 mile to the junction with US 50 heading east, then drive 0.7 mile to the Spooner Summit parking lot, on the north side of the highway. Entrance fees apply here as well.

Spooner Lake

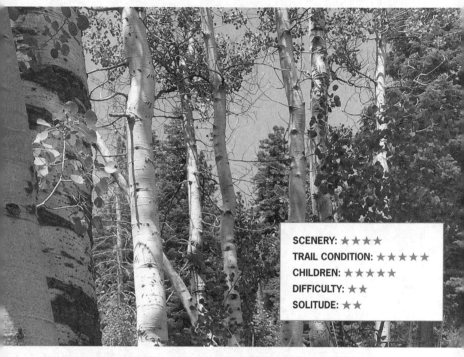

SCENERY: ★★★★
TRAIL CONDITION: ★★★★★
CHILDREN: ★★★★★
DIFFICULTY: ★★
SOLITUDE: ★★

A BEAUTIFUL ASPEN FOREST ADDS VISUAL AND AUDIBLE TEXTURE TO THE SPOONER LAKE TRAIL.

GPS TRAILHEAD COORDINATES: N39° 06.278′ W119° 53.817′

DISTANCE & CONFIGURATION: 3.4-mile balloon loop

HIKING TIME: 1–1.5 hours

OUTSTANDING FEATURES: Lakeside benches make great spots to enjoy the wildlife, wildflowers, aspen groves, and some fishing.

ELEVATION: 7,172′ at trailhead

ACCESS: Year-round; $10 entrance fee April 15–October $15, $7 otherwise

MAPS: *Tahoe Rim Trail* (Tom Harrison Maps)

FACILITIES: Pit toilet

COMMENTS: Dogs must be leashed on the trail.

CONTACT: Lake Tahoe Nevada State Park, 775-831-0494, parks.nv.gov/parks /marlette-hobart-backcountry

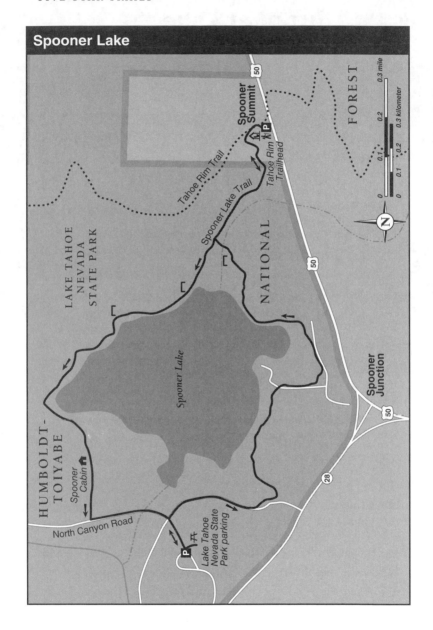

Spooner Lake

Overview

Embark from the Tahoe Rim Trail's Spooner Summit Trailhead to descend through an aspen grove on the way to the lake loop. If you're in a contemplative mood or hanker to watch birds, benches are well placed around the lake to accommodate you.

Route Details

Your slow walk around this former millpond will be rewarded with glimpses of wildlife—both fauna and flora. The trail is off-limits to bikes, but dogs on leashes are welcome.

Spooner Lake is one of those areas around Lake Tahoe that you're just as likely to visit in winter as in any other season due to the popular groomed trails and overnight cabins. If you like to trek on terra firma, though, this happens to be one of the areas that melts out soonest, allowing you to hike in late May or early June. Spooner Lake, along with Marlette Lake and Hobart Reservoir, was part of the famous Hobart-Marlette Water System that supplied Virginia City and the nearby mines. Spooner's former status as a millpond has been erased, and it's now known more for nature observation and winter recreation.

Start at the Tahoe Rim Trail (TRT) Trailhead at Spooner Summit. Here at the summit, Spooner's Hotel was a thriving business

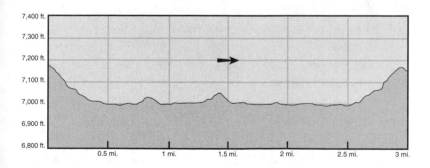

during the logging and mining heydays. Many wagons and their teamsters gathered here, crowding the narrow road. By 1915, Spooner's Summit had become a collection of ramshackle buildings, evidence of which has been erased from the scene. Alternately, you can park and begin your loop hike from Lake Tahoe Nevada State Park (LTNSP), about halfway around the lake.

Under cover of lodgepole and Jeffrey pines, take a moment to read about the area's natural history and the route of the TRT. For a more intrepid hike, leave this trailhead early in the morning and reach Tahoe Meadows by early evening. Pick up a TRT map for some additional details on that route.

A longer hike than Spooner Lake, albeit not as far-reaching as the TRT, is the hike to Marlette Lake described on page 56.

Walk along the TRT about 100 feet to the Spooner Lake access trail, then turn downhill to the left. Follow this shaded path west under lodgepole and Jeffrey pines, and enter the first of many groves of aspen as your trail turns northwest. The Basque sheepherders would use these smooth-barked trees as canvases for carving their initials, names, and pictures. You'll notice that Valentine's Day and birthdays are commemorated quite often (if you get a chance to read a few tree trunks away from the trail).

As you descend through the lush foliage, you will pass by the turnoff to Spooner Lake's south trail to the left. The sign will remind you that your dog must be leashed at all times while you are on the Spooner Lake Trail. Comfortable park benches have been placed off the path at frequent intervals around the lake and offer hikers a spot to relax with either a lake or mountain vista. You'll pass anglers of all ages, as Spooner Lake has a healthy population of lake trout.

Heading around the north side of the lake, you'll pass by the North Canyon Trail after 1 mile of footwork. The trail sign on the right, marked North Canyon Road, leads off uphill to the northwest. Turning right here leads uphill to Marlette Lake. Your route continues left around the west side of the lake. The open terrain here is pleasant under sunny skies because you can always cool off when you start uphill under the trees. About 100 yards south through the trees leads you to an interpretive display prepared by LTNSP. The parking area for LTNSP is about 300 feet west of here and can be reached via the trail.

Traverse south and turn east just after crossing a dirt road (leading to a locked gate at NV 28). The trail stays a respectful distance from the lake, always tucked just inside the trees, coming too close to the road before veering away. In a matter of minutes, you will reach the junction with the connector trail back uphill. This is a most beautiful section of trail, with several species of ferns, lilies, and an occasional snow plant in early season. In the fall, the aspens glow red and gold in the sunlight.

If you have time to sit and observe the wildlife, arrive very early and take a position on the south side of the lake. From here you may observe goshawks or owls as well as see signs of martens, raccoons, and possibly mountain lions.

Directions

From Carson City, drive south on US 395 to US 50 West, then 9 miles to the parking lot on the north side of the highway at Spooner Summit. Space here is limited; a fee is required to park.

From Incline Village, drive 10 miles south on NV 28 to the junction of US 50. Head east on US 50 and drive 0.7 mile to the Spooner Summit parking lot, on the north side of the road.

If the Spooner Summit parking area is full, you can park at LTNSP. It's on the east side of NV 28, 0.7 mile northwest of the US 50/NV 28 junction. Entrance fees apply here as well.

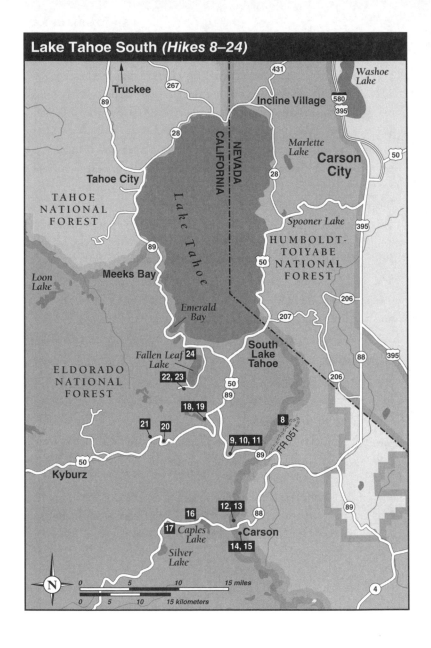

Lake Tahoe South *(Hikes 8–24)*

Lake Tahoe South

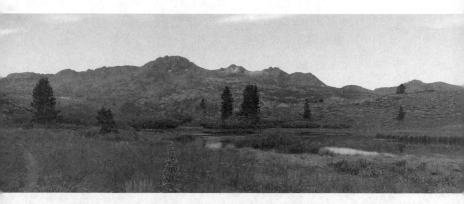

ROUND TOP AND THE SISTERS LOOKING SOUTH FROM ABOVE CARSON PASS
(see Hike 12, Carson Pass to Echo Summit, page 92)

8 # Freel Peak

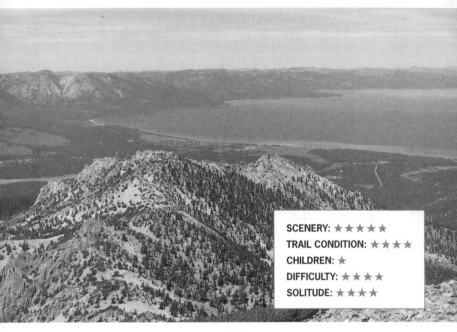

SCENERY: ★ ★ ★ ★ ★
TRAIL CONDITION: ★ ★ ★ ★
CHILDREN: ★
DIFFICULTY: ★ ★ ★ ★
SOLITUDE: ★ ★ ★

ALMOST EVERYTHING IS IN SIGHT FROM FREEL PEAK'S FLANKS, BUT SOUTH LAKE TAHOE COMES IN VIEW NICELY.

GPS TRAILHEAD COORDINATES: N38° 49.818′ W119° 54.047′

DISTANCE & CONFIGURATION: 10.2-mile out-and-back

HIKING TIME: 6–7 hours

OUTSTANDING FEATURES: This moderately strenuous hike will reward intrepid hikers with basin-to-range vistas from the highest peak in the Lake Tahoe region.

ELEVATION: 8,261′ at trailhead

ACCESS: Depends on snow

MAPS: *Lake Tahoe Basin* (Trails Illustrated 803)

FACILITIES: None

COMMENTS: Carry water.

CONTACTS: Humboldt-Toiyabe National Forest, Carson Ranger District, 775-882-2766, www.fs.usda.gov/htnf; US Forest Service, Lake Tahoe Basin Management Unit, 530-543-2600, www.fs.usda.gov/ltbmu

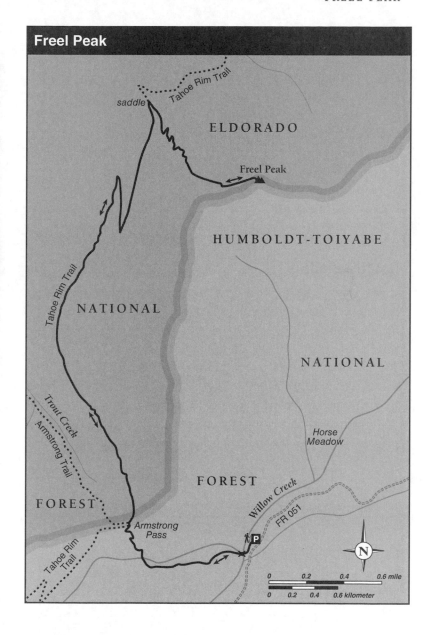

Overview

Traversing the path of the Tahoe Rim Trail (TRT) from Armstrong Pass to the saddle below Freel Peak is the "moderate" portion of this hike. The final mile to the summit is strenuous—if only moderately so—but the vista is breathtaking. Freel Peak, 10,881 feet above sea level and the highest peak in the Lake Tahoe region, is named for James Freel, who squatted on land at the base of the peak formerly known as Bald Mountain. Freel Peak serves as the easternmost summit of the Sierra. If peak-bagging is your thing, Jobs Sister and Jobs Peak are within easy reach of Freel Peak's summit and make excellent additions to this hike for hikers with long legs and extra energy.

Route Details

The trail begins on the other side of the bridge crossing Willow Creek, heading west from the clearing where you've parked. The bridge is now blocked by boulders, but this was formerly an off-highway-vehicle (four-wheel-drive) trail, once labeled with a non-bullet-ridden sign as Forest Road 051. Nothing to see here; keep moving. Walk on this track to a point 0.5 mile west of the bridge where, according to the sign, motorized vehicles must go no farther.

From here, where your singletrack begins by following the sign pointing to the TRT, it's less than 0.5 mile to Armstrong Pass. There, the Armstrong Trail coming up from Fountain Place (near the end of Fountain Place Road out of Meyers) joins the TRT coming from Big

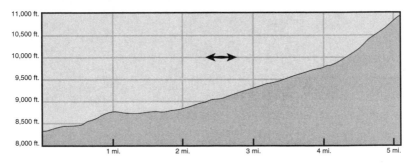

Meadow 9 miles to the southwest or from Star Lake 5 miles in the opposite direction. On the way to Armstrong Pass, you'll cross a small runoff stream as you swing around the spur of the ridge. Then your track along the TRT will traverse north on the west slope of the ridge.

Knowing that your destination is some 2,000 feet above you, there is no comfort in your brief descent through scattered boulders before you resume ascending. If you start within an hour of sunrise, your vista of South Lake Tahoe ahead will be spectacularly interrupted by the triangular shadow of your destination as it is silhouetted on the forest below.

About 1 mile from Armstrong Pass, the jutting rock outcrop called Fountain Face looms over your right shoulder as you tread steadily uphill through sagebrush, paintbrush, and rabbitbrush crowding and coloring your trail. This rock slab has nothing to attract serious climbers, and anyone else should stay on the trail to reach a more worthwhile destination. But Fountain Face is useful as a marker, because it's 1 mile ahead of the only switchback on this traverse. It's also 2 miles from the saddle below Freel and 3 miles from the summit.

Navigation is just plain easy on this distinct, mostly sand track bordered by rocks. Following footprints is about as difficult as it gets on this track. But following the correct set of footprints is fairly important in the upper section of this hike.

TRT volunteers deserve kudos for their efforts along this uphill path as it knifes through the shade of fir and pine. After a brief direction change to the south, your trail resumes its northward ascent to the saddle at just over 9,700 feet. On the way, in close succession, you'll cross three runoff streams that create a cool, verdant slope sporting larkspur, lupine, columbine, paintbrush, corn lilies, and assorted white and yellow flowers.

At the saddle, odd-shaped rock outcrops; trees gnarled and bent by the wind (the krummholz effect); and sparse, ground-hugging plant life are part of the interesting landscape, where you can also look out on Lake Tahoe. A sign to the south indicates that you are

1 mile (actually only 1,151 vertical feet) from Freel Peak. Depart the TRT at this point, and head south uphill through the trees.

Scree, gravel, and sand bordered by boulders, whitebark pine, and chasms make up the steep but distinct trail to the summit. Plenty of rock steps have been laid to help you up in the steepest sections. About two dozen switchbacks help you ascend this southerly track to the top. Sensitive plant areas are marked—right next to steep drop-offs. Don't tread on either. Mark these points in your mind so that you're prepared for them on your return. The sand underfoot slides easily on the rock here. After you cross the 10,000-foot mark, the steepness abates and the trail traverses an open scree slope east–southeast toward the summit.

At the top, a quarter-circle of stacked stone breaks the wind for tired hikers. Look among the rocks for the current peak register, which is now housed in an ammo can. In years past, communications antennas occupied the peak, but they have been removed, and only their foundations remain. Vistas into Lake Tahoe and the Carson Basin are interrupted only by Freel's companion peaks, Jobs Sister and Jobs Peak, which, as you can see from Freel, are within easy reach.

Directions

From the junction with US 50 in Meyers, drive south on CA 89. After the highway makes a looping turn to the east, you will see Big Meadow Trailhead on the left. Drive 4 miles east of Big Meadow Trailhead to the poorly marked junction with Willow Creek Road, where you'll leave the highway on poorly marked Willow Creek Road 4 miles east of Big Meadow Trailhead. Willow Creek Road is on the east side of CA 89 about 0.75 mile past Luther Pass. Willow Creek Road/FR 051 heads northeast toward Horse Meadow, where you can park.

Coming from Carson Pass or Carson City, Willow Creek Road is on the right, 1.75 miles north of the junction of CA 88 and CA 89 in Hope Valley.

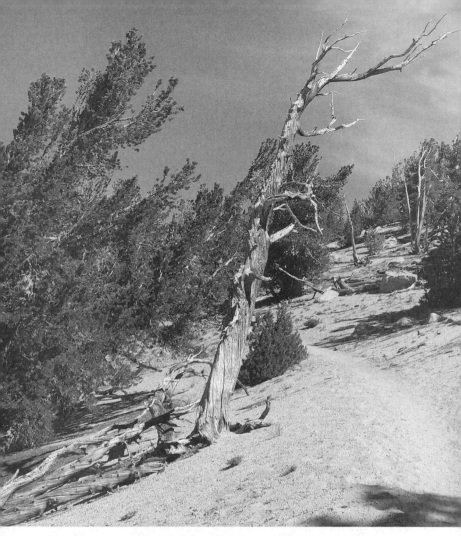

CHIN STRAPS REQUIRED ON THE WAY TO FREEL'S SUMMIT.

I advise that you use a high-clearance vehicle on this road, but careful driving in a wagon will also get you there. Drive 2.5 miles up FR 051 and cross Willow Creek on the bridge; then drive another 1 mile to cross a second bridge. Park in the open area east of the creek. A small wooden bridge across the creek is blocked by boulders. And so you've reached your parking spot. From here, you'll hike 0.5 mile to the trailhead.

Dardanelles Lake

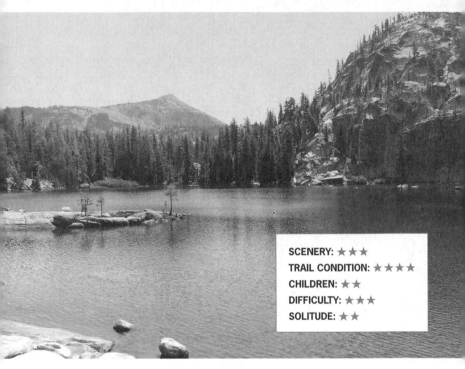

SCENERY: ★★★
TRAIL CONDITION: ★★★★
CHILDREN: ★★
DIFFICULTY: ★★★
SOLITUDE: ★★

A VARIED SHORELINE MAKES FOR SOME SECLUDED PICNIC SPOTS AROUND THE NORTH SHORE OF DARDANELLES LAKE.

GPS TRAILHEAD COORDINATES: N38° 47.318′ W120° 00.046′

DISTANCE & CONFIGURATION: 8.2-mile out-and-back

HIKING TIME: 2 hours

OUTSTANDING FEATURES: A small lake with lots of granite shoreline on which to sun, swim, picnic, and camp

ELEVATION: 7,263′ at trailhead

ACCESS: Year-round

MAPS: *Lake Tahoe Basin* (Trails Illustrated 803)

FACILITIES: Pit toilet

CONTACTS: Eldorado National Forest, Amador Ranger District, 209-295-4251, www.fs.usda.gov/eldorado; US Forest Service, Lake Tahoe Basin Management Unit, 530-543-2600, www.fs.usda.gov/ltbmu

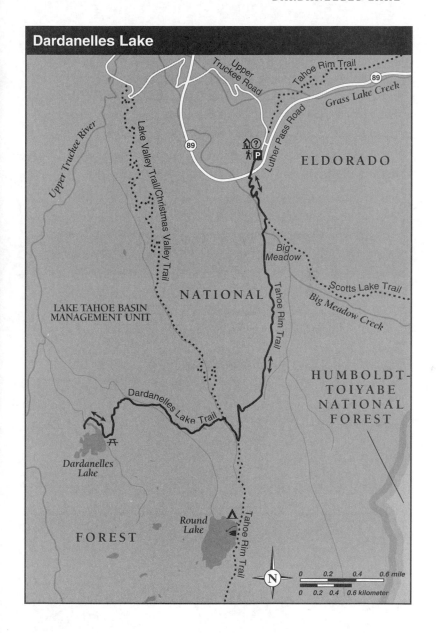

Dardanelles Lake

Upper Truckee Road

Tahoe Rim Trail

89

Grass Lake Creek

Luther Pass Road

Upper Truckee River

Lake Valley Trail/Christmas Valley Trail

89

ELDORADO

Big Meadow

Scotts Lake Trail

NATIONAL

Big Meadow Creek

Tahoe Rim Trail

LAKE TAHOE BASIN
MANAGEMENT UNIT

HUMBOLDT-
TOIYABE
NATIONAL
FOREST

Dardanelles Lake Trail

Dardanelles
Lake

FOREST

Round
Lake

Tahoe Rim Trail

N

| 0 | 0.2 | 0.4 | 0.6 mile |

| 0 | 0.2 | 0.4 | 0.6 kilometer |

Overview

Hiking on the Tahoe Rim Trail (TRT) means an outstanding trail and even better scenery. Begin with Big Meadow itself, a broad, flower-filled meadow where flowers, grasses, and trees are visibly and audibly alive with insects, birds, and small mammals. End with a refreshing dip in a beautiful mountain swimming hole.

Route Details

Meiss Country is the area between CA 88 and CA 89, from Echo Summit to Hope Valley. It's named after the Meiss family, whose father, Louis Meiss, emigrated from Germany to Drytown in the early 1840s. He built a cabin and pastured cattle on land about 1 mile west of Meiss Lake in the late 19th century. Meiss Country includes seven pleasant lakes nestled in a broken and jumbled geologic terrain where volcanism and tectonics combine to add to the Sierra stew.

The trailhead is located at the south end of the Big Meadow parking lot. An interpretive sign at the trailhead will give some insight as to the flora and fauna that you can expect to see along the trail. Any alerts or cautionary notices will be placed here. Continue walking south about 600 feet before a careful crossing of CA 89, where you regain the trail.

After just 0.6 mile and an elevation gain of 260 feet, you'll wade through the willows protecting Big Meadow Creek. The duff-and-granite

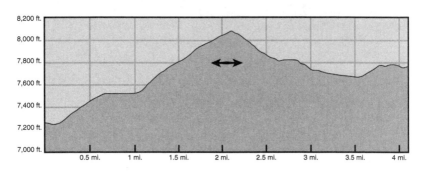

trail ascends with the help of switchbacks through lodgepole pine and incense cedar, punctuated by displays of lupine and Indian paintbrush. Granite outcrops surrounding the trail are used as steps more than once as the trail meanders close to the creek.

Just before crossing the creek, your trail is interrupted by the junction of the path to Scotts Lake leading to the left, while your trail, marked TO MEISS MEADOW, leads to the right. In that direction, the trees part and Big Meadow appears. If you have it with you, this is the last safe point to apply your insect repellent. On the positive side, your rapid arm waving can also be interpreted as friendly greetings to other hikers.

Big Meadow is about 2,000 feet long and almost half as wide, and its grassy acreage is ringed by pine and fir forest. Large erratics—geological masses that succumbed to gravity as their particular glacier melted—dot the meadow's landscape and provide small islands of solitude for day hikers. Less visible but ever present, these huge rocks seem more plentiful in the forest than the meadow.

Buttercups, columbine, and explorer's gentian flash yellow, crimson, and purple in the sun as the shadow of one lone cloud drifts across the meadow. Yellow warblers flash and sing while they dart around the edge of the meadow, probably chasing one of the thousands of butterflies that swarm the flowers. Why these birds aren't mosquito eaters isn't in the nature guide.

Under a warm sun and cobalt-blue sky, Big Meadow Creek gurgles through an S-curve, its fluid rhythm jamming with the trill of the "cheeseburger bird" (mountain chickadee) and the hums and clicks of bees, grasshoppers, and crickets. The instantly memorable symphony is recallable on the chilliest winter evening. Hold that thought.

Reaching the trees at the south end of Big Meadow, the trail narrows and begins ascending for the next mile. Your climb is steady and consistently southward over the roots and rocks gracing the trail. A handy set of 28 wooden stairs lends a vertical assist up through the lodgepole pines and white firs. You can see the red tops of snow plants bursting through the soil beside the trail.

Your ascent abates at about 2 miles along, where you start to notice some downed timber. The sandy trail then skirts an aspen grove that looks as if it has been subjected to the penknives of artistic explorers. While not exactly a meadow, this open area is exposed to the sun, which draws out the corn lilies by the thousands as soon as the snow melts. Insect repellent is a definite plus on this hike, especially along this section next to the creek.

At about 8,100 feet in elevation, you'll begin a short break from the climbing while you descend some easy switchbacks for the next 0.25 mile until you reach a junction with the trail to Dardanelles Lake via Lake Valley Trail, also known as Christmas Valley Trail. Here you will take a 180-degree turn northwest and hike 0.2 mile to the Dardanelles Lake Trail at the next junction.

Turn west, down and over one creek and then another one with boulders to assist your crossing. This packed-duff trail follows the creek 0.5 mile northwest through Western juniper, lodgepole pine, and some white fir before turning southwest. Take advantage of boulders once more at another stream crossing before beginning 0.35 mile of scenery and your final uphill to the eastern shore of Dardanelles Lake.

This deceptively small lake seems to have a generous amount of shoreline and flat granite bivy space around and on the north end's small peninsula. There are also some superb sites on which to picnic or camp above the lake on the east and northeast perimeters.

Directions

From US 50 in Meyers, turn south on CA 89 and drive 5.3 miles to the Big Meadow Trailhead parking lot on the left side of the road. It has pit toilets and water spigots, but no trash receptacles. The trailhead is at the south end of the lot. Turn left past the pit toilets and drive straight toward the trailhead.

Coming from Carson Pass or Carson City, take CA 88 to CA 89 north and drive 5.9 miles north to the Big Meadow Tahoe Rim Trail Trailhead on the right.

Round Lake

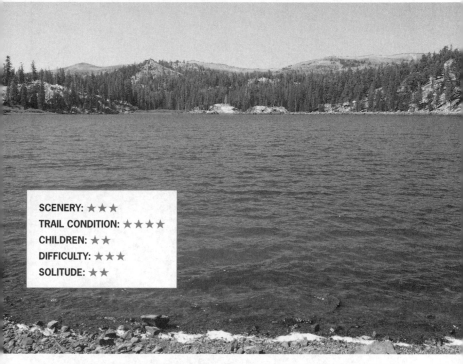

SCENERY: ★ ★ ★
TRAIL CONDITION: ★ ★ ★ ★
CHILDREN: ★ ★
DIFFICULTY: ★ ★ ★
SOLITUDE: ★ ★

ROUND LAKE IS RUMORED TO HAVE FISH, AND ANGLERS HAVE BEEN SEEN THERE.

GPS TRAILHEAD COORDINATES: N38° 47.318′ W120° 00.046′

DISTANCE & CONFIGURATION: 6.6-mile out-and-back

HIKING TIME: 2 hours

OUTSTANDING FEATURES: A walk through a lush montane meadow provides a pleasant start and easy access to a good fishing lake.

ELEVATION: 7,263′ at trailhead

ACCESS: Year-round

MAPS: *Lake Tahoe Basin* (Trails Illustrated 803)

FACILITIES: Pit toilet

CONTACTS: Eldorado National Forest, Amador Ranger District, 209-295-4251, www.fs.usda.gov/eldorado; US Forest Service, Lake Tahoe Basin Management Unit, 530-543-2600, www.fs.usda.gov/ltbmu

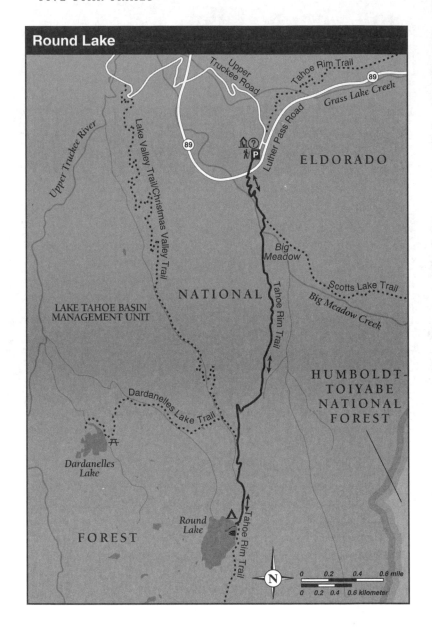

Round Lake

Overview

This moderate hike along the Tahoe Rim Trail (TRT) leads through a broad, flower-filled meadow to a placid lake reflecting a snowcapped peak in the background. The trail to this popular destination rises swiftly from the trailhead to Big Meadow, which is a destination in itself for many people. Other hikers, joggers, equestrians, and anglers continue a gentler ascent through this mixed-conifer forest to aptly named Round Lake.

Route Details

Meiss Country is an area bounded by CA 88 and CA 89, from Echo Summit to Hope Valley. It's named after Louis Meiss, who settled on land about 1 mile west of Meiss Lake. Meiss Country includes seven pleasant lakes nestled in a broken and jumbled geology where volcanism and tectonics combine to add to the Sierra stew.

The trailhead is located at the south end of the Big Meadow parking lot. An interpretive sign at the trailhead will give some insight as to the flora and fauna that you can expect to see along the trail. Any alerts or cautionary notices will be placed here. Continue walking south about 600 feet before crossing CA 89 where you regain the trail.

A series of switchbacks helps you up the 225 feet that it takes to reach Big Meadow, just 0.5 mile away. The duff-and-granite trail

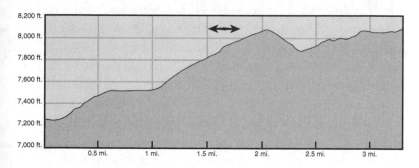

ascends under lodgepole pine and incense cedar, punctuated by displays of lupine and Indian paintbrush. Granite outcrops that surround the trail are used as steps more than once as the trail meanders close to Big Meadow Creek.

After the trail levels out, you'll encounter a junction where the trail to Scotts Lake leads to the left and our trail, marked TO MEISS MEADOW, leads to the right. In that direction, the trees part and Big Meadow appears. If you have it with you, this is the last safe point to apply your insect repellent.

A walk in any direction in Big Meadow yields a feast of activity and color from an abundance of sources. The meadow itself is some 2,000 feet long and perhaps half as wide and is ringed by pine and fir forest. The trees on the southwest margin are flanked by rock, which seems to hold snow long after the rest has vanished. Large erratics (geological masses that succumbed to gravity as their particular glacier melted) dot the meadow's landscape and provide small islands of solitude for day hikers. Less visible but ever present, these huge rocks seem more plentiful in the forest than the meadow.

Buttercups, columbine, and explorer's gentian flash yellow, crimson, and purple in the sun as the shadow of one lone cloud drifts across the meadow. Yellow warblers flash and sing while they dart around the edge of the meadow, probably chasing one of the thousands of butterflies that swarm the flowers. Why they aren't eating any of the millions of mosquitoes isn't in the nature guide.

Under a warm sun and cobalt-blue sky, Big Meadow Creek gurgles through an S-curve, its fluid rhythm jamming with the trill of the cheeseburger bird (mountain chickadee) and the hums and clicks of bees, grasshoppers, and crickets. The instantly memorable symphony is recallable on the chilliest winter evening. Hold that thought.

When the trail reaches the trees at the south end of Big Meadow, your trail will narrow and begin ascending for the next mile. Despite some roots and rocks in the trail, the climb is steady and consistently southward. A handy set of 28 wooden stairs will give you a vertical assist as you head up through the lodgepole pines and white firs. While you're looking down at your feet, glance to the side of the trail to see the red tops of snow plants bursting through the soil.

Just about the time the downed timber becomes noticeable, your ascent will moderate somewhat as the trail turns sandy and you start to skirt an aspen grove that looks as if it has been used as a Valentine's card. While not exactly a meadow, this open area is exposed to the sun, which draws out the corn lilies by the thousands as soon as the snow melts. Insect repellent is a definite plus on this hike, especially along this section next to the creek.

At about 8,000 feet in elevation, you'll begin a short break from the climbing while you descend some easy switchbacks for the next 0.25 mile until you reach a junction with the trail to Dardanelles Lake via Lake Valley (also known as Christmas Valley). If you want to go to Dardanelles, take a 180-degree turn north and hike about 1.5 miles to the lake. Your trail continues straight south, climbing gentle switchbacks about 0.5 mile through boulders of conglomerate rock. The trail walks up to a small rise overlooking Round Lake. Take any of the descending trails along the north end of the lake.

The rock closest to the lake—not friendly for sitting on—is conglomerate that has likely been sloughed off Stevens Peak and blown about in various andesitic eruptions. Despite the lack of smooth granite to relax on, numerous fishing spots dot the north and east shores. The lake's outlet is on the northwest shore and feeds the Upper Truckee River. As you walk over to the outlet, lodgepole chipmunks will begin following you for the easy meal. As cute as they are, resist the urge to feed them anything, for both their well-being and yours. Squirrels and chipmunks not only can become dependent on handouts, but they also carry the flea that transmits the plague virus. Keep your distance from them despite their cuteness. You will also be harried by Steller's jays—another famous camp robber, like Clark's nutcracker without the loud caw. With avian flu having been found throughout the foothills, it would be prudent to avoid sharing food with them, as well.

The TRT continues past the eastern margin of the lake 2.5 miles, south past Meiss Lake, to its junction with the Pacific Crest Trail. There, the TRT turns north toward Echo Summit. Round Lake is well known for its fishing, and that may be reason enough to tarry at this pleasant bowl of water. Retrace your steps for an easy hike out.

Directions

From US 50 in Meyers, turn south on CA 89 and drive 5.3 miles to the Big Meadow Trailhead parking lot on the left side of the road. It has pit toilets and water spigots, but no trash receptacles. The trailhead is at the south end of the lot.

If coming from Carson Pass or Carson City, take CA 88 to CA 89 North and drive 5.9 miles north to the Big Meadow Tahoe Rim Trail Trailhead on the right.

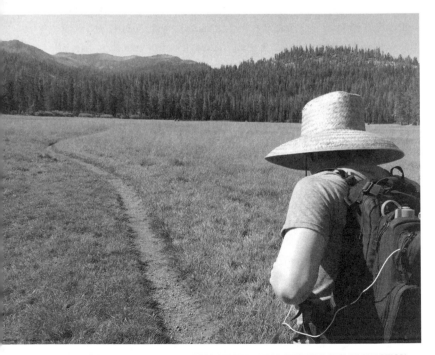

HIKES SOUTH FROM THE BIG MEADOW TRAILHEAD REQUIRE SUN PROTECTION.

Big Meadow to Kingsbury South

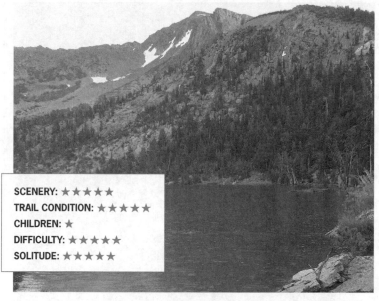

SCENERY: ★★★★★
TRAIL CONDITION: ★★★★★
CHILDREN: ★
DIFFICULTY: ★★★★★
SOLITUDE: ★★★★★

Photo: Jonathan Marsh

STAR LAKE IS A WELCOME SIGHT FOR THIRSTY TAHOE RIM TRAIL HIKERS.

GPS TRAILHEAD COORDINATES: N38° 47.419′ W119° 59.983′ (Big Meadow),
N38° 57.630′ W119° 53.230′ (Kingsbury South)

DISTANCE & CONFIGURATION: 23.8-mile point-to-point with shuttle

HIKING TIME: 12 hours

OUTSTANDING FEATURES: The route traverses lush forests of mixed conifers, passes
several meadows thick with wildflowers, climbs within easy reach of the highest peak in the
Lake Tahoe Basin, and offers incredible vistas of the basin's peaks and ranges.

ELEVATION: 7,325′ at trailhead

ACCESS: Year-round

MAPS: *Tahoe Rim Trail* (Tom Harrison Maps)

FACILITIES: Pit toilet

CONTACTS: Eldorado National Forest, Amador Ranger District, 209-295-4251,
www.fs.usda.gov/eldorado; Humboldt-Toiyabe National Forest, Carson Ranger District,
775-882-2766, www.fs.usda.gov/htnf

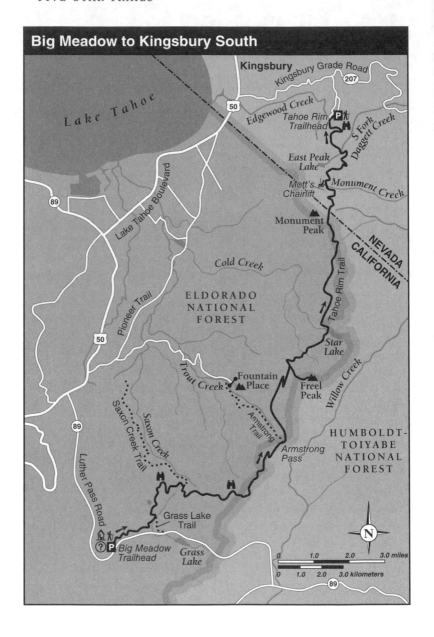

Big Meadow to Kingsbury South

Overview

Flat becomes but a memory when you embark from Big Meadow. Gain about 1,500 feet in the first 5 miles. Then the trail turns north and begins to climb up to a high point of about 9,725 feet at the base of 10,881-foot Freel Peak, the highest peak in the Lake Tahoe Basin. Views along the way span from Round Top in the south to the Pyramid Peak and the Crystal Range in the west to Lake Tahoe in the north. Eastern vistas of the Carson Range pop in and out of view as you mostly descend to some degree or other all the way to Heavenly Valley.

Route Details

Leave the trailhead kiosk and begin your eastward trek up this serpentine trail. The path is pleasant and nicely shaded by red fir and Jeffrey pine. You gain elevation just to keep above CA 89, which you roughly parallel for about 1.5 miles. Turn north, entering switchbacks, and continue climbing. After 2 miles on the trail, look for the junction with the trail to Grass Lake, 1 mile away. As you snake up this slope, watch for vistas to the south when the trees break. Cross a stream on some well-placed logs in this aspen-flocked glade.

Springwater emerges from beneath a large rockfall of granite boulders in a ravine about halfway up to the vista on the ridge. Your

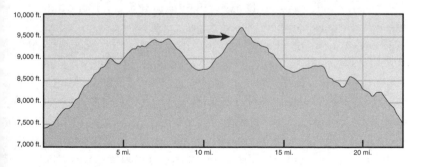

view from this spot is to the east and southeast. Once you make the ridge, just before turning east, look for a superb vista overlooking the airport and Lake Tahoe's south shore.

From that vantage point, head southeast and climb to a tiny saddle between two small knobs. For the first time in about 5 miles, you begin to descend. Switchback down to the junction with the Saxon Creek Trail before you start ascending once again. Climbing northeast, look right to see a meadow heavy with color. The trail stays away from this one but climbs to the fringe of a grassy meadow on the far side of the knoll. The trail slides around to the right and heads uphill.

If you need more flowers, Freel Meadows waits for you less than 100 feet uphill. Corn lily, aster, Indian paintbrush, wallflower, lupine, elephant's head, and larkspur display themselves at the height of summer. The sand-and-gravel trail skirts the verdant swale and 5 minutes later is out of sight as the trail curves away, downhill through the boulders.

Walk uphill through scattered lodgepole to another magnificent vista point. Lake Tahoe spreads out to the northwest, and Hell Hole Canyon sits 1,000 feet below your perch. To the south are Round Top and Elephants Back, while Freel Peak stands on the northeastern horizon. This view stays with you as you cross the broad, open slope heading east. Swing around the wooded knoll and start tracking high above Willow Creek, northeast toward Armstrong Pass.

Continue north and the trail emerges from behind its windbreak and makes for the exposed ridgeline. Note the stout lodgepole pine in krummholz configuration. Red fir joins lodgepole and Western white pine as you leave this barren landscape and descend toward Armstrong Pass, 700 feet below. Pass the trail marked for the Oneidas Street Trailhead, and continue northeast toward Freel Peak and then Star Lake, 5 miles ahead.

Begin the assault on the Freel massif by, uh, descending through scattered boulders; then enjoy a slightly uphill traverse to the north. As you walk through sagebrush and rabbitbrush about 1 mile after Armstrong Pass, you'll pass the rock outcrop called Fountain

Face. After another mile, you'll reach the only switchback before the saddle, which is yet another mile distant.

Bordered by rocks, the sandy trail uses only these two direction changes on its way to the high point of about 9,725 feet. On the way, you'll have a chance to water up at three runoff streams in close proximity to one another. The water and lush foliage here create a cool environment complete with the scents of lupine, larkspur, corn lily, columbine, and assorted white and yellow flowers.

Resume the northward climb along this immaculate trail (kudos to Tahoe Rim Trail Association volunteers) to reach the saddle, where you're only 1,150 vertical feet from Freel Peak—which, at 10,881 feet, is the highest point in the basin. It may not be the day to do it, but hiking to the peak is a worthwhile trip that you will enjoy having done. Although, tagged onto a 23-miler, it might make for a busy day.

Descend northwest and sharply adjust east, continuing to hike down past Freel to the foot of Jobs Sister. When you're about 0.75 mile past the saddle, watch for a small runoff stream. If you need good campsites, ascend this small stream for bivy options. Lose about 500 feet and cross a rock-filled ravine before making the final descent to Star Lake's outlet stream. The slope offers excellent views of Lake Tahoe in the distance and small meadows below.

The most rewarding aspect of Star Lake is its ice-cold foot soak. But it's a great place to fill up on water, too. Make sure to do your water-getting away from the foot-soaking. The campsites close to the lake are good for a siesta, but better choices lie above the lake's northeast corner, away from the trail and lake. After a relaxing break, make a dogleg north, then west, to jog over the ridge spur. Then resume the northward descent through pine and hemlock forest, and repeat the maneuver in 0.75 mile. Follow the trail as it traverses high above High Meadows on its 3.4-mile leg to Monument Pass.

Though initially steep, the trail's descent moderates some as the trees thin and views to the west open up. Pyramid Peak stands out beyond Tahoe and the Crystal Range. Your vista changes as you reach Monument Pass, where you'll have a vista of Carson Valley and Jobs Sister; it's only fitting as you'll enter Nevada just 10 minutes ahead. At this point, you will leave the Eldorado National Forest and enter the Humboldt-Toiyabe National Forest.

Curl-leaf mountain mahogany and buckwheat occupy this dry, boulder-ridden pass. The sandy trail descends steeply toward Mott Canyon. The steep slopes and drastic elevation difference along this narrow, exposed section of trail may induce a case of the mountain willies as you traverse beneath Monument Peak. Enter and exit one canyon and then another. In the second one, you'll find Mott Canyon chairlift hanging motionless above Mott Canyon Creek. This is your first indication of your long approach to Heavenly Valley Nevada ski area.

Climb out of the canyon's shade on a steep, sandy utility road for a gain of 230 feet in 0.5 mile. Traverse north across slopes well treed with lodgepole and Western white pine. Make a looping descent across a bowl just below East Peak Lake, and traverse to a crossing of its outlet, South Fork Daggett Creek. Pass under another chairlift, and in about 0.5 mile your descent to Heavenly will begin in earnest. Round a pointy knob and begin to switchback down to the resort. Watch for a park bench, which is situated nicely for contemplative gazing.

Manzanita and tobacco brush are interspersed with Jeffrey pine and fir as you descend the obvious trail. A trail marker at the end of the second switchback identifies the Tahoe Rim Trail and lists mileages to all the sites you hiked past. Continue downhill another 0.5 mile to the Stagecoach parking lot and a well-deserved hopped beverage.

Directions

To reach the Big Meadow Trailhead from South Lake Tahoe, drive 4.8 miles on US 50 to Meyers. Turn left onto CA 89 and drive 5.3 miles south to the Big Meadow parking lot, on the left. You'll find pit toilets and water, but no garbage services, at this large parking area. Overnight camping is allowed. Turn left at the entrance and drive

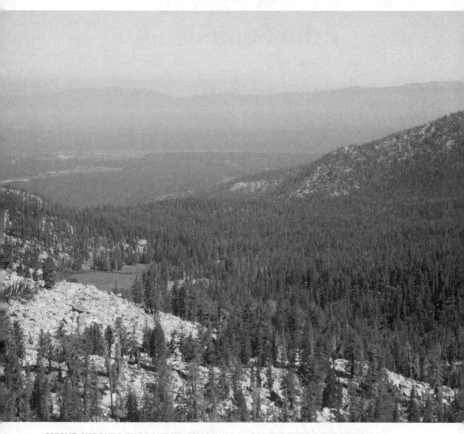

SMOKE SHROUDS THE LAKE WHEN VIEWED FROM THE TAHOE RIM TRAIL.

slowly downhill to park. The trailhead is at the TRT kiosk about 500 feet north of the pit toilets.

Leave another vehicle at Daggett Pass. From South Lake Tahoe, drive 5.6 miles north on US 50, through Stateline, and turn right onto NV 207. Drive 3.1 miles to Tramway Drive and turn right. Drive 1.7 miles to the Heavenly Valley Stagecoach Lodge parking area. Leave your ride near the Stagecoach chairlift and look for the Tahoe Rim Trail kiosk west of the lot, near the large boulders.

Carson Pass to Echo Summit

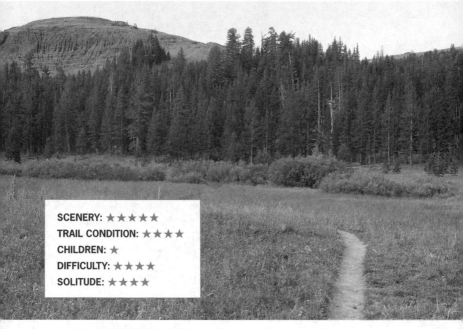

SCENERY: ★★★★★
TRAIL CONDITION: ★★★
CHILDREN: ★
DIFFICULTY: ★★★
SOLITUDE: ★★★

IN THE UPPER TRUCKEE RIVER BASIN

GPS TRAILHEAD COORDINATES: N38° 41.804′ W119° 59.525′ (Carson Pass),
N38° 48.740′ W120° 01.990′ (Echo Summit)

DISTANCE & CONFIGURATION: 13.5-mile point-to-point with shuttle

HIKING TIME: 8–9 hours

OUTSTANDING FEATURES: Vistas into the Upper Truckee River drainage; memorable
wildflower displays; volcanic, granitic, glaciated terrain

ELEVATION: 8,546′ at trailhead

ACCESS: Year-round; $5 parking fee

MAPS: *Lake Tahoe Basin* (Trails Illustrated 803)

FACILITIES: Toilets, water

CONTACT: Eldorado National Forest, Amador Ranger District, 209-295-4251,
www.fs.usda.gov/eldorado

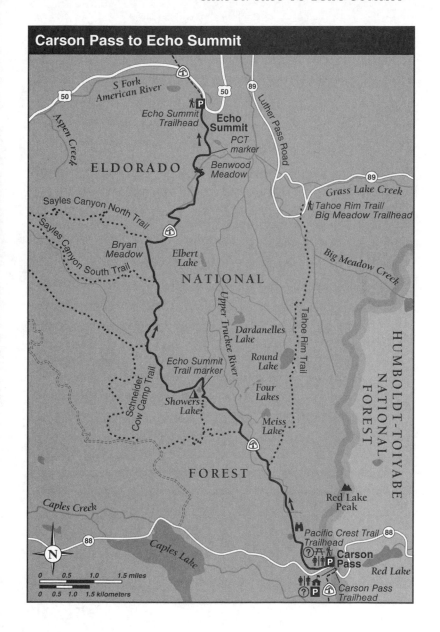

Carson Pass to Echo Summit

Overview

Day hiking these three classic trails is a five-star scenic experience worth every bit of effort. However, it isn't triple the work—in this case, it's the pleasure that is multiplied. The Pacific Crest National Scenic Trail (PCT) isn't called "scenic" for naught. And there just weren't any shabby trails used when creating either the Tahoe Rim Trail (TRT) or the Tahoe–Yosemite Trail (TYT).

Leave historic Carson Pass and travel northwest into the Upper Truckee River basin, which is bound by volcanic ridges from Stevens Peak in the northeast, Red Lake Peak to the southeast, and Little Round Top to the south. The basin includes many lakes (remnants of the glaciers that occupied the area): Meiss Lake, Four Lakes, Round Lake, Dardanelles Lake, Showers Lake, and Elbert Lake.

The high elevation point comes as you emerge from the cirque beneath Little Round Top. From there it's downhill, more or less, through small meadows and over steep trail to your goal near the Desolation Wilderness.

The grass-filled meadows and rock-laden hillsides are chock-full of iris, lupine, larkspur, paintbrush, corn lily, blue flag, bluebell, sulfur flower, Chinese houses, mule's ears, elephant's-head, buttercup, leopard lily, penstemon, and many more wildflowers still than I could identify.

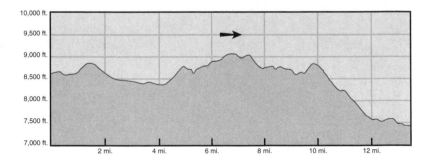

Route Details

Reorganize your gear for the last time at the picnic table, and then head initially west on the sandy, lodgepole-clad trail. Keep to the left of the outcrops to round the ridge at the foot of Red Lake Peak. Traffic sounds fade in about 0.5 mile as your hike north is interrupted only by a few quick switchbacks on this treeless, south-facing slope. Hike north again, uphill toward a small pond where a solitary nearby tree provides much-needed shade after the climb. From this saddle, follow the distinct trail north through iris and paintbrush to an obvious vista point in the middle of this sloping meadow about 1.5 miles from the trailhead.

The Upper Truckee River basin and Lake Tahoe lie in front of you. They are bordered by mountains consisting of metamorphic and sedimentary rock along with intrusive igneous rock in the form of granitic plutons like Half Dome. All of this has, from time to time, been overlain with volcanic debris, which, itself being somewhat soft, has been eroded by water and ice. Glaciers have occasionally entered the scene, dropping debris of one sort, called erratics, randomly around the terrain. At other times, these rivers of ice tidy up after themselves, pushing their leftovers into neat piles called moraines which take form either to the sides as lateral moraines or in front which is left behind as a terminal moraine. Your trail undulates across the northwest foot of Red Lake Peak, steadily descending above but alongside the creek.

About 1.75 miles from the pond and after a few honest crossings of the nascent Upper Truckee River, you can spot a side trail that leads west over to the two cabins on the river built by Benjamin Meiss early in the last century. To this point, you've been on the PCT and TYT only. The next junction just ahead is the bottom turn on the TRT; to the right, it leads 2 miles east to Round Lake, with Big Meadow another 3 miles farther on. Your destination's trail is ahead to the left through the beautiful Upper Truckee Meadows. Showers Lake, 2 miles distant, makes a great lunch spot, while Bryan Meadow, 6 miles on, will only slow you down with all the wildflowers. It's about 11 miles from this TRT junction to Echo Summit.

Moments after joining the TRT, the track widens and again crosses the headwaters of the Upper Truckee River. Your vistas through the Upper Truckee Meadow are spectacular. At the final crossing, the trail resumes its normal width and heads through willows up into the pines. After a long, level stretch leading past Meiss Lake and crossing Dixon Canyon, the trail turns into an up-ramp that gains about 375 feet in nearly 0.75 mile. On this hill to Showers Lake, you'll again be treated to a walk through shoulder-high clusters of wildflowers. A fair campsite sits above the lake on the left, with better sites under nice tree cover along the eastern shore, especially at the north end.

A trail junction at the north end of Showers turns you to the right, away from the lake toward Echo Summit. Walk to the right of the marker about 150 feet, and look for the faint trail that steeply descends another 100 feet to cross the lake's outlet stream. A sharp U-turn will send you packing southwest under an imposing granite wall. A fairly gentle ascent on a sandy trail carries you up to boulder city, where a lupine-dominated meadow follows a copse of lodgepole pines. Heading into the cirque beneath Little Round Top, the northbound trail continues its upward trend, and the wildflower viewing becomes more like wading. You will absolutely wallow through dense stands of Sierra willow, giant lupine, larkspur, Indian paintbrush, and plenty more. The color extravaganza starts on the volcanic overhangs above the trail and reaches down to the exposed granite below the trail. With snow lingering on the north-facing slopes beneath an azure sky, the scene is spectacular.

Impromptu bivy sites can be found north of Little Round Top, at around 8,900 feet in elevation. Here, at this hike's high point of almost 9,000 feet, the vista of the cirque just crossed is massive. A rest here is a great idea. A quarter-mile hence, your sandy trail skirts

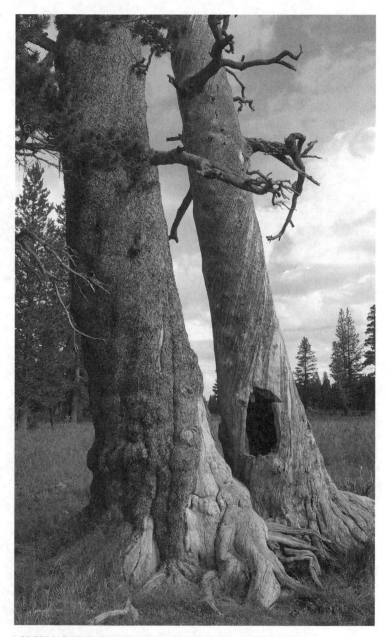

LODGEPOLE PINES PLAYING NEW ROLES IN THEIR LATER STAGES

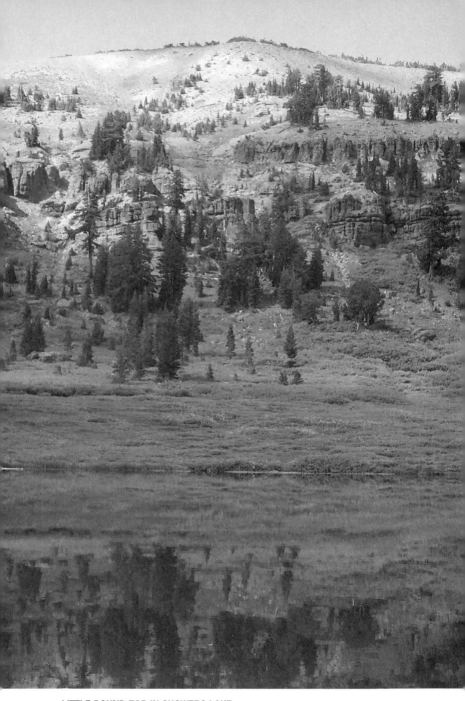

LITTLE ROUND TOP IN SHOWERS LAKE

a small meadow on its south side. Contour, more or less, to another small, heather-fringed meadow where the trail from Schneider Cow Camp intersects the PCT/TYT/TRT. Evidence of cattle operations is hard to miss around here. The sandy trail turns to rock when you pass the next meadow, ready to make a 350-foot descent through the lodgepole forest toward Bryan Meadow. In another 1.5 miles, you'll come to a junction for the trail leading west down Sayles Canyon to Sayles Flat Campground at US 50. Another trail junction 0.8 mile farther north, in Bryan Meadow, eventually leads to the same campground.

Lodgepoles crowd your trail, which passes Bryan Meadow and then departs the small saddle. From here, you face a tedious traverse across a heavily forested slope, followed by a steep descent to finish the route. When you reach the ridgeline, 0.75 mile from the saddle, your vista is into the canyon that you'll bounce down from ridge to ridge. Drop 150 feet in the next 0.25 mile into this small cirque, where you'll find an excellent bivy site to the right of the trail just above a flowing creek. Cross the creek and continue on the PCT, which makes tight switchbacks beneath impressive granite outcrops down the west side of the ravine. Use roots and rocks as stairs until you get to the crossing about 0.3 mile past the bivy site. Look for a bivy site on the right, above the creek. The route remains steep and boulder-filled, with cramped switchbacks alongside the steep slant of the ravine's walls. Trekking poles are more than valuable coming down this segment of trail. The slopes are pleasantly shaded by pine and fir, and pileups of boulders as big as Yugos fill the ravine in places.

Finally, when your creek is tame enough to be straddled by a footbridge, you're nearing Benwood Meadow, where scarlet fritillary (*Fritillaria recurva*) grows by the trail. The next stream crossing after the bridge is marked by a lodgepole pine scarred with a blaze. No beeline for the PCT, though. First walk west, then north; then dip east before you're past the meadow, climbing away to the northwest through manzanita and boulders. Continue your downward traverse under cover of mixed conifers.

At the PCT–TRT marker in a clearing, you should be able to see your final destination, which is just beyond the buildings at the snow park. Trail signs will lead you the final half mile, down the west slope of the snow park, keeping above and passing the large parking lot. Continue up the trail, watching for signs for the PCT, TRT, and Pony Express Trail as you walk north.

Directions

After coffee at Alpinas in South Lake Tahoe, take US 50 south 4.7 miles to Meyers, then turn left on CA 89 and drive 11.2 miles to CA 88 in Hope Valley. Turn west (right) on CA 88 and drive 8.7 miles to Carson Pass, where there is a ranger station and large parking lot with toilets on the south side of the road. Get maps and information here and, most important, purchase a season-long parking pass for $25—or pay $5 for every night you're parked.

The parking lot for this hike's trailhead is 0.3 mile west, on the north side of CA 88. Equipped with toilets (often much cleaner than the ones at the ranger station), trash receptacles, and water, this parking area accommodates horse trailers. The trailhead for the PCT on this side of Carson Pass is located at the northwest corner of the parking lot, where a picnic table sits opposite an information kiosk. Pass the parking-fee receptacle on your way to this trailhead.

The trailhead at the Echo Summit end is 8.8 miles south of South Lake Tahoe on US 50, just 0.2 mile past the highway maintenance station on the right. Turn left at Echo Summit Sno-Park, where there's room for a dozen cars in the trailhead lot. (Don't park in the large lot at the snow park.) The trail's terminus is on the right, in the trees just above the parking area. There are no facilities at this trailhead. Pit toilets are located inside the snow park but may not be available year-round.

13 # Showers Lake

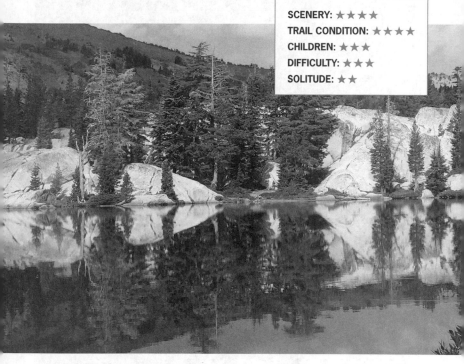

CALM MORNING AT SHOWERS LAKE

GPS TRAILHEAD COORDINATES: N38° 41.804´ W119° 59.525´

DISTANCE & CONFIGURATION: 10.6-mile out-and-back

HIKING TIME: 8 hours

OUTSTANDING FEATURES: Pacific Crest Trail, Tahoe–Yosemite Trail, and Tahoe Rim Trail; flower-filled meadows; granite peaks; historic cabins; pristine lake; vistas over the Upper Truckee River to Lake Tahoe

ELEVATION: 8,546´ at trailhead

ACCESS: Year-round; $5 parking fee

MAPS: *Lake Tahoe Basin* (Trails Illustrated 803)

FACILITIES: Pit toilets

CONTACTS: Eldorado National Forest, Amador Ranger District, 209-295-4251, www.fs.usda.gov/eldorado; US Forest Service, Lake Tahoe Basin Management Unit, 530-543-2600, www.fs.usda.gov/ltbmu

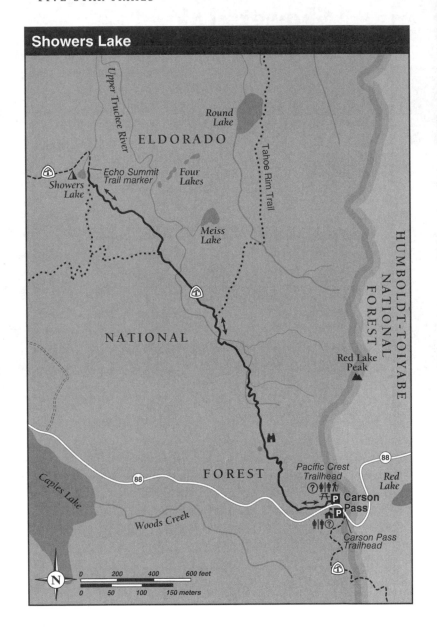

Showers Lake

Round Lake

ELDORADO

Upper Truckee River

Echo Summit Trail marker

Showers Lake

Four Lakes

Tahoe Rim Trail

Meiss Lake

NATIONAL

Red Lake Peak

HUMBOLDT-TOIYABE NATIONAL FOREST

FOREST

Pacific Crest Trailhead

Carson Pass

Red Lake

Caples Lake

88

Woods Creek

Carson Pass Trailhead

N

| 0 | 200 | 400 | 600 feet |
| 0 | 50 | 100 | 150 meters |

Overview

Hiking on this section of the Pacific Crest and Tahoe Rim Trails simplifies your day hike, because the path is well maintained and well signed, and the uphills and downhills are fairly easy. You won't need extensive navigational skills (although you should always carry a map and compass and know how to use them) to find your way along this trail heading north into the Upper Truckee River drainage. Keep your camera ready, because you'll discover plenty of vistas and wildflowers along the way. To protect the meadows, stay put to look at the original cabins on the edge of Meiss Meadow; they're easily viewed from the trail. This is a great hike for families with children able to handle a light pack. There is little shade for much of the hike, so take plenty of water (or a method to treat it) and wear appropriate sun protection.

Route Details

The Carson Pass Trailhead, a pleasant waypoint on the Pacific Crest Trail (PCT), is found at the west end of the parking lot behind the bushes and parking-fee receptacle. Rest your backpack on the picnic table while you read information about the PCT on the kiosk. If you have aspirations for a long hike, you can see that this trail will take you more than 1,000 miles south to Mexico or more than 1,500 miles north to Canada.

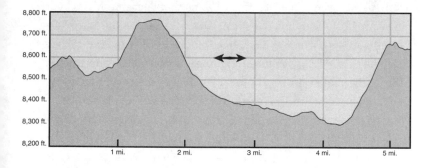

This hike is a simple 5 miles to Showers Lake. It begins by heading west, climbing at a moderate rate, to round the spur of Red Lake Peak on a sandy and rocky trail. Weary long-distance hikers might find some comfort in a couple of impromptu campsites in the first 0.5 mile. (The closest water, however, is an intermittent stream another 0.5 mile north.)

A moderate 300-foot climb up a south-facing slope takes you up to a former cattle pond. According to a US Forest Service biologist, the giardia count has been reduced significantly in this area since cattle have been restricted. This pond is now an acceptable water source for hikers, but better streams are not far ahead. If you're tired from the exposed hike, the tree on the east side of the trail is a welcome sight. While you rest here, get your camera out, because the vistas and the wildflowers over the next 0.5 mile are spectacular.

The almost level trail invites lingering to take pictures of giant lupine, corn lily, woolly mule's ear, mountain bluebell, Indian paintbrush, larkspur, penstemon, aster, sticky cinquefoil, elephant's-head, and Sierra stickseed. This easy section of trail is about 100 feet above the canyon floor and gradually descends to the meadow over the next 0.75 mile. You'll cross a few reliable runoff streams as you come abreast of the western flank of Red Lake Peak. Shortly, your view down to the northeast will be filled with Meiss Meadow and Lake.

An impromptu trail leads west (but, to protect the meadow, don't use it) over to the site of the cabins that Benjamin Meiss built in about 1901 when he settled this section of land, 1 mile from the lake that bears his name. The Tahoe Rim Trail (TRT) and the Tahoe–Yosemite Trail (TYT) join the PCT at the junction 500 feet northwest. This is the southern turn on the TRT, almost the beginning of the TYT, and not quite the midpoint of the PCT. If you're glad that yours is only a day hike, just continue left on this multi-appellation trail 2 miles to Showers Lake. The route right leads hikers northeast 2 miles to Round Lake, where bears have been known to steal food.

Soon the trail turns into a doubletrack while heading across the meadow, which is soggy in early season. You will cross and recross the nascent Upper Truckee River until the doubletrack runs out after your last creek crossing. The trail leads through willows and climbs into white fir trees above the meadow.

Your route continues northwest while rising about 400 feet to a point above the southeast corner of the lake. Before you drop down to the lake, notice the wind-protected campsite on the west side of the trail with a view over the lake. There are some highly impacted sites right next to the lake just after you descend to it. Better sites— and good swimming—can be found among the lodgepole, fir, and hemlock around the east and north sides of the lake. From this vantage point, you have a good view of Little Round Top as it looms just 1 mile to the west.

If you're continuing toward Echo Summit on the PCT, your trail follows the east shore to the lake's outlet, then crosses to the south to navigate around a solid granite wall. Older maps show a trail around the south side of the lake, but this area is marshy and the trail has faded from view.

Directions

From the junction of CA 88 and CA 89 in Hope Valley, drive 9 miles west on CA 88 to the parking lot on the north side of the road, 750 feet west of the Carson Pass Information Station. From the west, turn left into the lot 3.95 miles east of the Kirkwood Junction on CA 88. This lot and the lot on the south side at Carson Pass are the only legal places to park, and the daily fee is $5. (These parking areas have pit toilets, trash receptacles, and often water.) If you're staying overnight, you'll need to pay for two days of parking. An annual pass, available at the Carson Pass Information Station for $25, can be used at other trailhead parking areas in the Eldorado National Forest and the Lake Tahoe Basin Management Unit, which are described elsewhere in this book. *Hint:* If you hike even a few times each season in the Lake Tahoe Basin, this is a good pass to purchase.

Fourth of July Lake

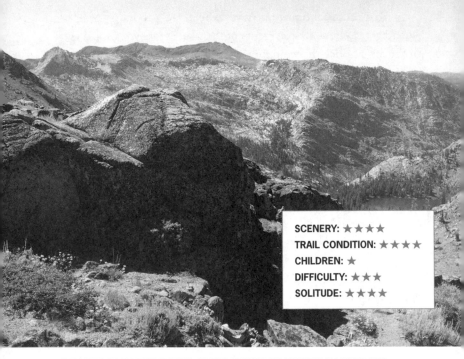

SCENERY: ★ ★ ★ ★
TRAIL CONDITION: ★ ★ ★ ★
CHILDREN: ★
DIFFICULTY: ★ ★ ★
SOLITUDE: ★ ★ ★ ★

BIG VISTA FROM THE FLANKS OF THE SISTERS TO FOURTH OF JULY LAKE

GPS TRAILHEAD COORDINATES: N38° 41.673′ W119° 59.364′

DISTANCE & CONFIGURATION: 12.2-mile out-and-back

HIKING TIME: 8 hours

OUTSTANDING FEATURES: Botanical displays everywhere; wide vistas in every direction; solitude at camp; huge view down Summit City Creek′s canyon

ELEVATION: 8,580′ at trailhead

ACCESS: Year-round; $5 parking fee

MAPS: *Mokelumne Wilderness* (US Forest Service)

FACILITIES: Pit toilet

CONTACT: Eldorado National Forest, Carson Pass Management Area, 209-258-8606, tinyurl.com/carsonpass

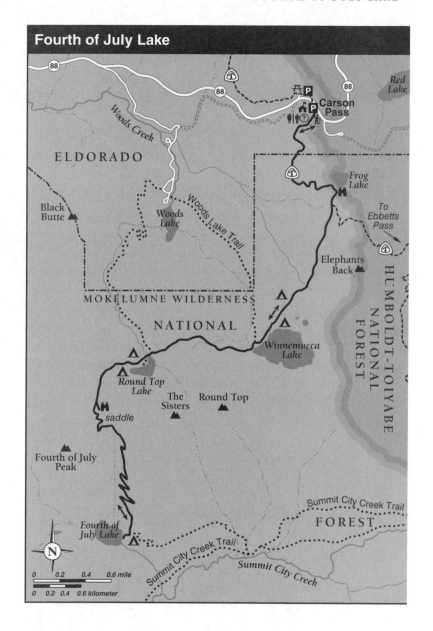

Fourth of July Lake

Overview

Enjoy the massive wildflower displays along the trail past Winnemucca and Round Top Lakes, and then leave the crowd behind as you trek to an isolated alpine tarn tucked beneath Fourth of July Peak, almost ready to drop into the Summit City Creek canyon. New trail improvements make this a simple and safe trek downhill.

Route Details

Embarking from the trailhead near the ranger station, the lupine-lined trail begins climbing at a nominal rate through lodgepole and fir. Stone stairs and switchbacks help the uphill effort along here. After crossing a few runoff streams and just 0.5 mile of easy walking from the trailhead, you'll enter the Mokelumne Wilderness. A tilted meadow where wildflowers begin their display for the senses follows your exit from the treed trail. This is a good time to remember where you packed the sunscreen.

Mingling with sagebrush, woolly mule's ears wave their yellow heads in the wind, accompanied by the crimson of paintbrush and the baby blue of Sierra stickseed. The trail is a visual delight to travel. A few more uphill steps send hikers past Frog Lake, just to the east of the trail. Elephants Back dominates the southern horizon just in front of you. It may not look exactly like a pachyderm from this vantage point, but to the immigrants coming from the

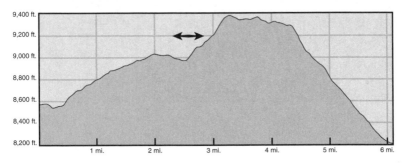

east in the mid-19th century, it seemed accurate down to the ivory tusk made of snow.

Turn from this behemoth, walking toward the more distant giant to the southwest—Round Top. Within 500 feet, the trail splits away from the Pacific Crest Trail, which heads southeast to Ebbetts Pass while you traverse this open slope full of Sierra iris and columbine on a wide, sandy trail. If you're lucky enough to time your hike with a recent rainfall, this slope will be packed with Indian paintbrush, larkspur, shooting stars, sticky cinquefoil, and fragrant lupine.

As you approach rockbound Winnemucca Lake, you'll pass some campsites on the left and right. Notice the marker posts indicating the number of each campsite. This system of impacting specific "sacrifice" sites repeatedly is a good way to prevent degradation of more-pristine areas. This method of campsite identification is also followed at Round Top Lake and Fourth of July Lake. Bypass any trails descending left to Winnemucca Lake; continue south and west for Round Top Lake.

Just before crossing the outlet stream from Winnemucca, walk past the junction for a trail that leads 2 miles down to Woods Lake, where there is a campground. Continue past the outlet and climb across the gnarled feet of Round Top. Take advantage of the runoff stream crossings where wildflower species—flax, Sierra primrose, elephant's-head, lavender gilia, and baby blue eyes—tend to congregate. The 300 vertical feet that you see straight ahead takes you about 0.5 mile to the overlook of Round Top Lake.

Pass a junction with another trail leading to Woods Lake, again 2 miles below and to the north, then cross the outlet stream on your way west. A sideways comma prostrate at the foot of Round Top (more accurately, it is below The Sisters), this tarn has a smattering of numbered campsites in the trees away from the lake. Avoid further impact to the areas right next to the shore by spending any idle time away from the water. The broad, sandy trail leads west around the last of The Sisters, where you enjoy good views before dropping into Fourth of July Lake's cirque.

When you round the westernmost hillside, a faint trail leads ahead to the left. That is a spur trail that comes to a stop overlooking Fourth of July Lake from the south side of The Sisters. Leave the lookout point and head southwest along the trail, directly into the saddle. Five switchbacks lower you about 250 feet before you make an eastward traverse of about 0.3 mile. You'll drop another 200 feet before changing direction midslope for another 0.3-mile traverse. The narrow trail is rocky but travels through crowds of colorful flowers, which are especially helpful in distracting hikers on their way out. After a couple of meltwater streams, the trail continues angling downhill. Don't be surprised if your destination looks tantalizingly close from this point. Another 20–30 minutes will take care of this vertical aberration.

After the trail's midpoint, five increasingly longer switchbacks control your descent. The lake is right there, but the trail seems to veer away to the east. This new trail avoids the final steep section that posed problems and kept many hikers away from this lake. The older, steeper trail is blocked off where the new trail swings away. Avoid using the closed section of trail: It's not faster, although it may be shorter.

Finally nearing lake level, your trail makes a circuitous approach, first southeast and then south, until you are even with the middle of the lake. At that point, a junction reveals a trail leading east, down-canyon to Summit City Creek, 800 feet below. Your trail leads west directly toward the lake for 200 feet, where you can begin finding markers for tent sites. At the lake's outlet 200 feet south, frigid water dives through the lodgepole and Western white pines on its way to Summit City Creek and, eventually, the Mokelumne River. The western shore, or rather the mountain containing it, is graced with some huge Jeffrey pines, sometimes in thick stands but often standing alone on a precarious mountain perch.

Your hike out is less difficult than it appears. It will take an average hiker about an hour of steady but slow hiking to exit this massive backcountry bowl.

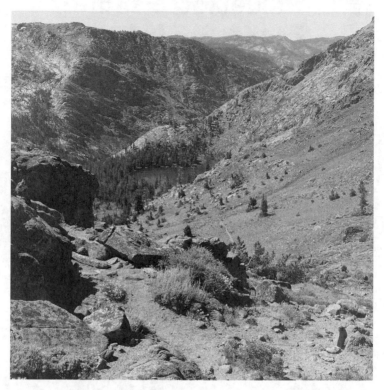

FOURTH OF JULY LAKE SITS LIKE A GEM 1,000 FEET BELOW YOUR LOOKOUT.

Directions

After leaving South Lake Tahoe, drive south on US 50 for 4.7 miles to Meyers, turn left on CA 89, and drive 11.2 miles to CA 88 in Hope Valley. Turn west (right) on CA 88 and drive 8.7 miles to Carson Pass, where there is a ranger station and large parking lot with toilets on the south side of the road. You can get maps and information here and, most importantly, you can purchase a season-long parking pass for $25—or pay $5 for every night you're parked here.

Overnight permits for this special-use area of the Mokelumne Wilderness are available only at this ranger station and on a first-come, first-serve basis. (See Appendix B, page 289, for more information.)

Winnemucca and Round Top Lakes

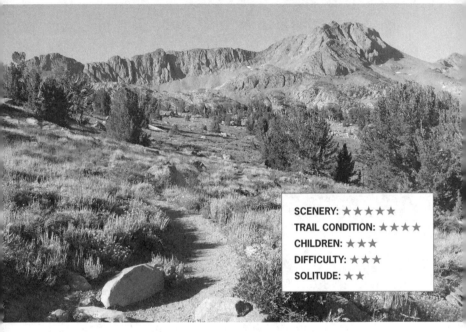

THE TRAIL TO ROUND TOP BOASTS RANDOM DISPLAYS OF FLOWERS.

SCENERY: ★ ★ ★ ★ ★
TRAIL CONDITION: ★ ★ ★ ★
CHILDREN: ★ ★ ★
DIFFICULTY: ★ ★ ★
SOLITUDE: ★ ★

GPS TRAILHEAD COORDINATES: N38° 41.673′ W119° 59.364′

DISTANCE & CONFIGURATION: 7.25-mile out-and-back

HIKING TIME: 4.5 hours

OUTSTANDING FEATURES: Two miles south of Carson Pass, these two subalpine tarns are easily reached by hikers of all ages, and they are great destinations for family overnights. While this is a popular area for day hikes, the only thing crowding this trail is wildflowers.

ELEVATION: 8,580′ at trailhead

ACCESS: Year-round; $5 parking fee

MAPS: *Mokelumne Wilderness* (US Forest Service)

FACILITIES: Pit toilet

CONTACT: Eldorado National Forest, Carson Pass Management Area, 209-258-8606, tinyurl.com/carsonpass

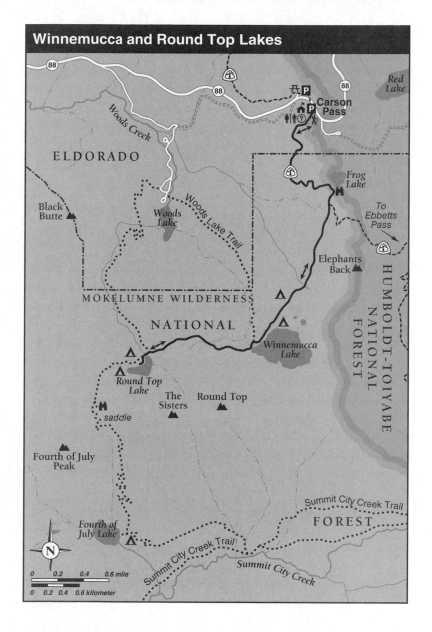

Winnemucca and Round Top Lakes

Overview

For the first mile to these easily accessible lakes, you may share your trail with Pacific Crest Trail (PCT) thru-hikers. Unfortunately, they will probably hurry on without enjoying the wildflower bonanza that day hikers have ahead of them. Within 2 short miles, you will see and smell the colors and scents of more than two dozen varieties of wildflowers. Bring your camera and field guide, along with plenty of insect repellent and sunscreen. Both lakes have several campsites, which are used by permit on a first-come, first-serve basis. While these campsites are "sacrifice" sites meant to minimize further human impact to the area, they are well placed, offering both seclusion and views.

Route Details

After you read about Snowshoe Thompson and Kit Carson at the historical monument adjacent to the parking lot, walk to the east end of the lot, where you can gain valuable information inside the ranger station. Your hike starts out at about 8,600 feet in elevation in the Eldorado National Forest before it quickly passes into the Mokelumne Wilderness and a specially protected zone. If you camp in this special-use area, ensure that you've received a permit and an assigned campsite from the ranger.

Begin with a short walk from the mileage sign adjacent to the ranger station. Your sandy and boulder-lined trail will start to gain

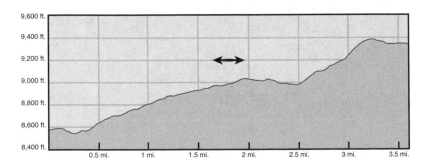

elevation just after passing the Carson Pass and PCT Trailhead sign. You'll immediately notice lupine adding color to the forested trail.

After you cross a rather lazy stream, begin traversing uphill to navigate around a large outcrop. Within 0.5 mile, you will enter the Mokelumne Wilderness. Your effort to traverse this mass of granite is assisted by steps intended for young knees. The elevation gain turns mellow, however, and even the final switchbacks up to Frog Lake are rather lazy.

After emerging from the forest onto a tilted meadow filled with woolly mule's ears, sagebrush, and Indian paintbrush, the trail rises to the level of Frog Lake, where, coincidentally enough, you'll find a convenient vista point. At your feet will be plenty of sticky cinquefoil and lavender gilia for your macro pictures. Off to the south are The Nipple and Round Top for your telephoto shots.

The trail turns away from this vista at 8,870 feet in elevation and runs slightly southwest toward Winnemucca Lake, which is about 1.3 miles away and sits at 8,975 feet. If you're looking at the ground and all of its color, it would be understandable if you missed the sign on your left indicating the junction where the PCT diverges and heads to Ebbetts Pass. Unless you're interested in an unplanned 22-mile hike, take the right-hand fork to Winnemucca.

Although you're hiking uphill, this sandy and broad trail makes the travel a bit easier. From this point you have a good view of Caples Lake to the west. In a few moments, the trail will become rockier, root-filled, and coincidently, a bit steeper. About this point, you may be glad that you applied sunscreen at the trailhead, because the trail is completely exposed except for scattered trees around the lakes.

As your trail continues to Winnemucca, you'll be astounded by the color flowing downhill from the surrounding rocks: scarlet subalpine paintbrush, Applegate's paintbrush, Torrey's lupine (plus three or four others), meadow penstemon, elephant's head, columbine, Sierra stickseed, mountain bluebell, giant mountain larkspur, meadow larkspur, shooting star, Western blue flag iris, Western blue flax, and Sierra primrose—and (if this hasn't whetted your appetite) there are more to discover.

Approaching Winnemucca Lake, you will descend from a gentle rise, where you'll see numbered campsites on both sides of the trail. If you're continuing to Round Top Lake, avoid the trails that descend to the left. But Winnemucca is a fine destination in itself. The large boulders (actually glacial erratics) around the lake make excellent wind-protected alcoves, secluded from other hikers, where you can enjoy a sheltered picnic.

Bypassing Winnemucca Lake, keep left at the trail junction, the first of two, with the Woods Lake Trail just before crossing Winnemucca's outlet stream on a well-anchored, stout log. Turn due west to begin a 450-foot climb to Round Top Lake, 1 mile away. You'll begin by crossing small runoff streams while traversing an alpine meadow sloping beneath Round Top. Mountain heather, Sierra primrose, and little stalks of elephant's head lead you uphill to a level area at the midway point of a steep meltwater runoff, which is crossed easily enough with the assistance of some well-placed rocks. The holdup, as usual, is the profusion of flowers crowding this junction: sky-blue flax, Sierra primrose, larkspur—all the usual suspects.

Whitebark pine, its male cones reddish purple and swollen with pollen, crowds the ground in its bent and dwarfed krummholz condition. Turn to face south and focus on the geology of Round Top and The Sisters to its west. Before you is layer upon layer of ancient ocean floor that has been lifted thousands of feet, altered by heat and pressure, turned, twisted, and carved by tectonic and glacial forces over eons. Round Top Lake, like Winnemucca, is a glacial tarn—the result of meltwater being contained by the lateral or terminal moraines created by the glacier. Before reaching Round Top Lake, you ascend to 9,450 feet in elevation, where you stand on a lateral moraine.

A short, steep descent will take you to a trail junction entering from the north, just next to the trees. This is the second of the two pack trails to and from Woods Lake, 2 miles away. The shade provided by these trees makes this spot a popular gathering place for hikers to

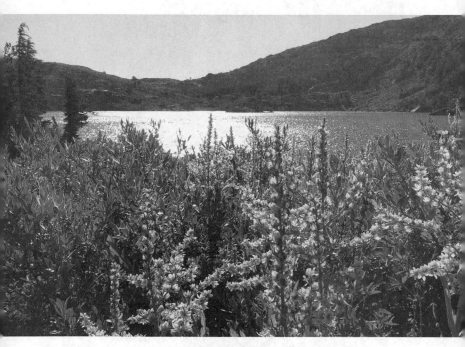

WINNEMUCCA LAKE CAPTURES THE MORNING SUN.

exchange information and swap stories. If you're camping overnight here, cross over the lake's outlet stream and amble a short way to the numbered campsites on either side of the trail.

Directions

From South Lake Tahoe, drive south on US 50 to Meyers, and then turn left on CA 89. Drive 11.2 miles to CA 88 in Hope Valley, where you'll turn west and drive about 7.5 miles to Carson Pass. Trailhead parking is on the south side of the highway. You can purchase a parking permit for $5 per day or $25 per season. No permit is required for day hikes, but you must have one for overnight camping (see Appendix B, page 289, for more information). Overnight parking requires two day fees.

Lake Margaret

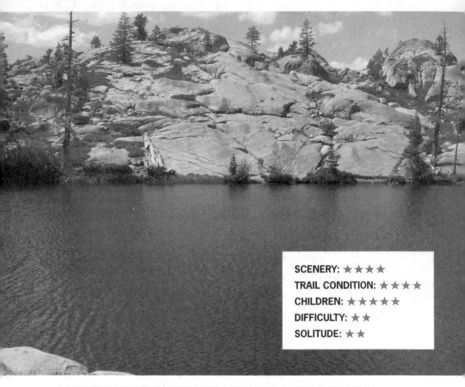

SCENERY: ★ ★ ★ ★
TRAIL CONDITION: ★ ★ ★ ★
CHILDREN: ★ ★ ★ ★ ★
DIFFICULTY: ★ ★
SOLITUDE: ★ ★

DIMINUTIVE LAKE MARGARET OFFERS ROOM FOR A VERY CHILLY SWIM.

GPS TRAILHEAD COORDINATES: N38° 42.258´ W120° 04.175´

DISTANCE & CONFIGURATION: 4.8-mile out-and-back

HIKING TIME: 2.5 hours

OUTSTANDING FEATURES: Pristine, jewel-like lake at the end of a well-defined, moderately easy, picturesque trail

ELEVATION: 7,747´ at trailhead

ACCESS: Year-round; $5 parking fee

MAPS: USGS *Caples Lake*

FACILITIES: Pit toilet

CONTACT: Eldorado National Forest, Amador Ranger District, 209-295-4251, www.fs.usda.gov/eldorado

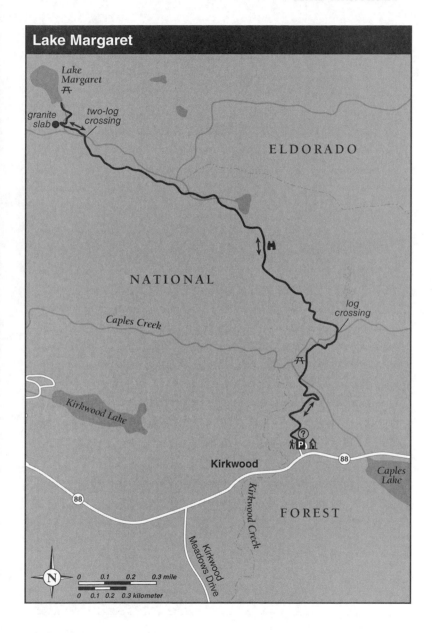

Overview

Lake Margaret is nestled amid a sloped granite field north of Kirkwood Lake. On this 2.4-mile descending traverse, you'll cross Caples Creek twice and will be able to enjoy the flowers that crowd these small, wet meadows. No navigation skills are needed to follow this highly blazed trail, allowing you to concentrate on children's questions along the way. The dirt-and-duff track mostly stays under the lodgepole, with a few short intervals on granite. Rockbound and dainty, Lake Margaret shines in the bright sun, inviting picnickers and swimmers.

Route Details

From the trailhead you zigzag downhill, losing 130 feet in 0.4 mile only to regain the majority of it a few thousand feet later. On your gentle descent, the sandy and rocky trail crosses the roots of white fir and lodgepole pine. You may notice a blaze in the form of a small *i* on trailside trees. In fact, if you were to start counting the blazes near the trailhead, you would reach 50 well before the lake. From a rocky overlook minutes away from the trailhead, you can hear the sound of Caples Creek below. In another few minutes, you'll cross your first branch of that creek. A sound log here makes for an easy crossing. You can see your trail ahead.

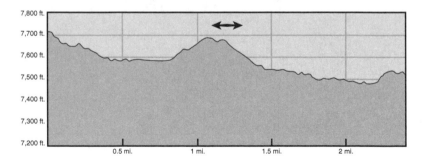

As the trail continues north, it is squeezed between the creek on the left and a small, domed outcrop on the right. If the ground is dry, you may find a couple of picnic spots among the lodgepole pines just as you approach this outcrop. You'll notice a casual trail going into the meadow just before your track turns east and meets willows lining the granite wall. Corn lilies, plentiful lupine, meadow penstemon, and asters grow among the fresh grass here.

Continue around the dome to the east, and parallel Caples Creek to a low, large log that reaches across the wannabe river. You're now 0.75 mile from the trailhead. After you cross, you'll return to a northwesterly course, again skirting a small meadow where you can look back and see the wall of granite behind you.

Zig right and zag left at the trail signs that help you up some rocky steps at the end of this meadow. Watch for a directional sign painted on the boulder. There, you'll begin to climb the rocky trail heading northwest. Switchback up through the lodgepole, and by about the 1-mile point, your trail will begin to skirt another outcrop. Pass by the casual trails leading to the little pond, and follow the enormous blazes and ducks. Take a moment to look around from the vista point just above the little pond.

Now you begin descending this outcrop toward the north, where you have a view of pine- and fir-studded granite ahead of you. Follow the ducks through the S curves, and continue descending on a dirt path to the west that leads to a rocky chute and a descending sandy trail. Head to the left of the next meltwater pond.

The log causeway near the runoff stream just past this pond marks the 1.5-mile point of your route. A small meadow sits to the south, and the granite knob to the north.

Continue downhill on the lupine-lined duff trail adjacent to the creek. Wolf lichen sticks to the trees, and aspen leaves rustle in the slightest breeze. Indian rhubarb and corn lilies gather around the stream to make a huge display of green foliage.

At the next creek crossing, head to the right of the trail to use the double-log arrangement that heads straight into a thicket of Indian rhubarb and willows. Crash through and continue on your sandy trail northwest.

A trail sign sends you east, up to the wall of a granite outcrop where some well-placed ducks lead straight up across the granite to the north. Descend to Lake Margaret with a slight water view on your way. The trail will lead you around to the lake's east side, which has some nice picnic spots. You'll also find some up on the rock above the lake to the east or to the south.

Directions

From the west, take CA 88 from Jackson 56 miles to the Kirkwood ski area. The turn into the Lake Margaret parking lot is 0.5 mile ahead on the left.

From South Lake Tahoe, take US 50 for 4.8 miles to the CA 89 turnoff in Meyers. Drive 11.2 miles south on CA 89 to CA 88, where you'll turn right (west). Lake Margaret's parking lot is 13.8 miles ahead, just past Caples Lake on the right. A parking fee applies.

The entrance is signed and the parking lot has room for about 20 cars. There are no facilities here, but there is a kiosk with local information posted at the trailhead.

Thunder Mountain

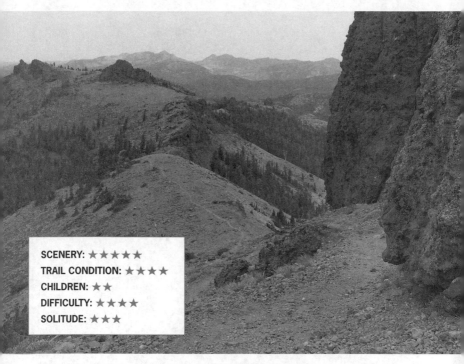

SCENERY: ★★★★★
TRAIL CONDITION: ★★★★
CHILDREN: ★★
DIFFICULTY: ★★★★
SOLITUDE: ★★★

VOLCANIC DEBRIS MARKS THE TRAIL TO THUNDER MOUNTAIN.

GPS TRAILHEAD COORDINATES: N38° 42.334′ W120° 06.439′

DISTANCE & CONFIGURATION: 7.8-mile out-and-back

HIKING TIME: 3.5–4 hours

OUTSTANDING FEATURES: Wildflowers covering sloped meadows; volcanic geology; wall-to-wall vistas from the summit

ELEVATION: 7,936′ at trailhead

ACCESS: Year-round

MAPS: USGS *Caples Lake*

FACILITIES: None

COMMENTS: Carry water.

CONTACT: Eldorado National Forest, Amador Ranger District, 209-295-4251, www.fs.usda.gov/eldorado

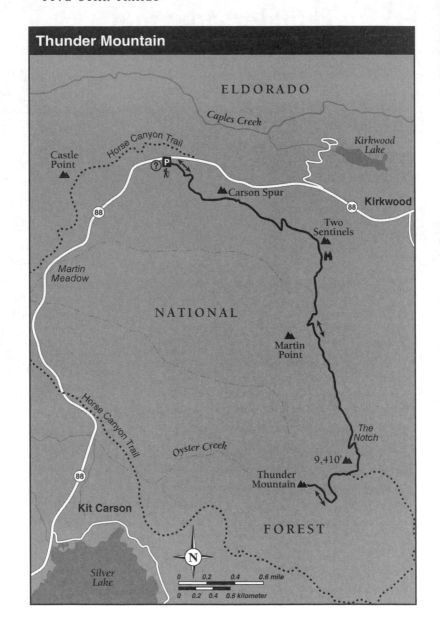

Thunder Mountain

ELDORADO

Caples Creek

Kirkwood Lake

Castle Point

Horse Canyon Trail

Carson Spur

88

88 **Kirkwood**

Two Sentinels

Martin Meadow

NATIONAL

Martin Point

The Notch

Horse Canyon Trail

Oyster Creek

9,410'

Thunder Mountain

88

Kit Carson

FOREST

N

Silver Lake

0   0.2   0.4   0.6 mile

0   0.2   0.4   0.6 kilometer

Overview

Look for a clear day to hike through this volcanic terrain up to spectacular vistas overlooking Silver Lake, the Mokelumne Wilderness, the Desolation Wilderness, and Kirkwood Meadows. The trail winds steadily up about 1,500 feet through huge, sloping meadows full of wildflowers and often thick stands of pine and fir. This hike takes you to Amador County's high point.

Route Details

Your easily identified trail embarks on a dirt path under cover of red fir and lodgepole pine. Enjoy their shade along with the lupine blues, paintbrush reds, and mule's ears yellows as you ascend and roughly parallel the road for a bit. Turn away from the road and begin climbing the forested slope. When you break out of the trees, you're greeted by a long, sloping meadow covered with woolly mule's ears accented with asters, lupine, and bright and profuse scarlet gilia. As you traverse the meadow and approach the snow-diversion panels atop Carson Spur's ridge, you can see the Two Sentinels ahead to the southeast and Martin Point to the south, with Martin Meadow and the setting moon far to the west.

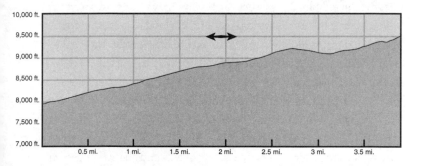

As you approach the ridgecrest, you'll encounter a unique pair of conifers—a Jeffrey pine and a Western juniper. Their stunted, misshapen, downhill branches shield their trunks, and their enormous lower branches reach the ground on the uphill slope, bracing themselves against the winds that often scream across this point.

As you briefly pass the avalanche control devices high above the highway, the tree cover thickens, and the trail soon resumes its steady uphill trudge. Your eastward march beneath the firs is interrupted by a couple of switchbacks that draw you closer to another avalanche-prone slope and more volcanic detritus. Layered lava on ashfall on lava flow, these remnants of eons of volcanism stand about 900 feet above the highway and tower over hikers on the trail. Turn southwest as you leave the Two Sentinels behind.

A beautiful vista opens both to the east and west after about 1.75 miles of uphill wandering. Silver Lake and Kirkwood Meadows spread beneath you on either side of the ridge. The trailside flowers now include dandelion and pussypaws, all being mauled by bees. At the next volcanic monster, the trail veers around to the right, where blue flax, pink primrose, purple penstemon, yellow wallflower, and red paintbrush are among the trailside color bursts.

Your southbound trail passes beneath Martin Point's eastern twin. Sierra gentian, lupine, and paintbrush join in as you make a beeline along the exposed ridge. The vistas here are, as you might imagine, incredible. But pictures and views may not be on your mind as you hike uphill in the wind past the Kirkwood ski resort's OUT OF BOUNDS signs, which warn skiers that rescue may be expensive if even possible. Aside from the views of Kirkwood, and far more dramatic, are the volcanic slopes to the west as you look over to 9,408-foot Thunder Mountain and the ghoulish-looking terrain beneath it.

Ahead, you can see The Notch, where the trail maneuvers west of a block of volcanic wreckage. After a brief but serious set of switchbacks to attain The Notch, the trail descends between two volcanic bombs and intersects with a casual trail leading uphill to a false summit at 9,360 feet.

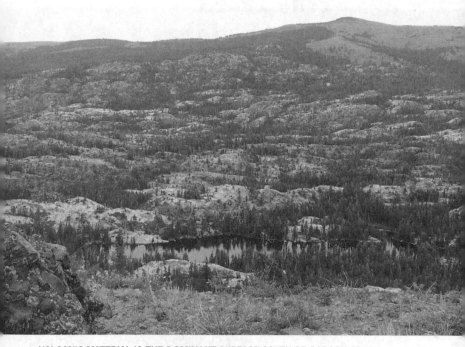

VOLCANIC MATERIAL IS THE DOMINANT SURFACE SOUTH OF CARSON SPUR.

Directions

Thunder Mountain's trailhead is 0.4 mile west of the Carson Spur on CA 88. Starting in South Lake Tahoe on US 50, drive 4.7 miles to Meyers, where you'll turn left onto CA 89. Drive 11.2 miles to the junction with CA 88 in Hope Valley. Turn west and drive 8.7 miles to Carson Pass, then continue west another 7.4 miles to the trailhead parking area, on the south side of CA 88.

If coming from the west, the trailhead is 3.2 miles east of the Kit Carson Lodge at Silver Lake or 54 miles from Jackson.

The dirt parking area supports about a dozen cars but has no other facilities. An informational kiosk with relative trail locations and distances is posted on the edge of the parking area. From there, you can easily see the trailhead in the southeast corner.

18 Echo Lakes to Lake Aloha

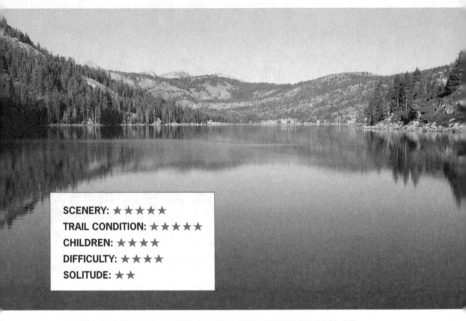

SCENERY: ★ ★ ★ ★ ★
TRAIL CONDITION: ★ ★ ★ ★ ★
CHILDREN: ★ ★ ★
DIFFICULTY: ★ ★ ★ ★
SOLITUDE: ★ ★

ECHO LAKE STANDS SERENE IN THE EARLY MORNING'S COOL AIR.

GPS TRAILHEAD COORDINATES: N38° 50.125′ W120° 02.664′

DISTANCE & CONFIGURATION: 15-mile out-and-back

HIKING TIME: 8 hours (overnight)

OUTSTANDING FEATURES: This hike features two famous trails alongside two of the most popular lakes in the Tahoe region. Easy access to a dozen more stunning lakes is eclipsed by the dazzling display of granite presented by the Crystal Range; towering overhead are Pyramid and Ralston, Price and Jacks, Cracked Crag and Echo Peaks.

ELEVATION: 7,425′ at trailhead

ACCESS: Depends on snow; permits required for day hiking and overnight camping

MAPS: *Desolation Wilderness* (Wilderness Press)

FACILITIES: Pit toilet

CONTACTS: Eldorado National Forest, Amador Ranger District, 209-295-4251, www.fs.usda.gov/eldorado; US Forest Service, Lake Tahoe Basin Management Unit, 530-543-2600, www.fs.usda.gov/ltbmu

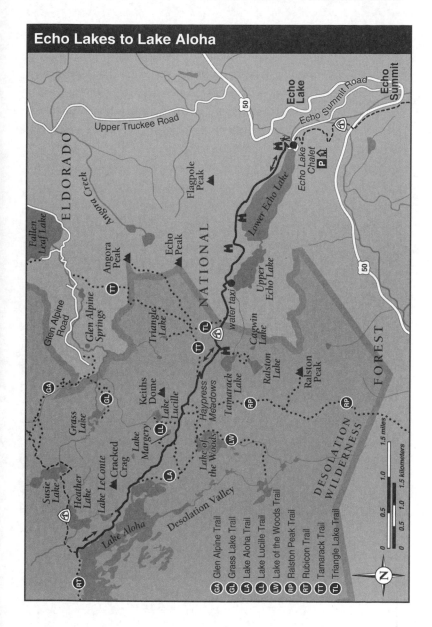

Echo Lakes to Lake Aloha

- **GA** Glen Alpine Trail
- **GL** Grass Lake Trail
- **LA** Lake Aloha Trail
- **LL** Lake Lucille Trail
- **LW** Lake of the Woods Trail
- **RP** Ralston Peak Trail
- **RT** Rubicon Trail
- **TT** Tamarack Trail
- **TL** Triangle Lake Trail

Overview

The Desolation Wilderness is one of the most visited backcountry areas in California. Because of its proximity to the Bay Area and Sacramento and its easily accessible trailheads, this entry to the Desolation Wilderness is always highly trafficked, so much so that there are daily quotas for overnight camping. Day hikers are asked to register at the trailhead or at a US Forest Service visitor center at no charge; overnight campers must pay to secure a permit. A good place to do that online is here: tinyurl.com/dwovernightcamping.

The trail to Lake Aloha presents no navigation challenges, although a compass and a map are essentials. Note that this trail has many intersecting trails. Fortunately, it's part of the Pacific Crest Trail (PCT) and Tahoe Rim Trail (TRT), and that means great signage for hikers.

This hike leads you to the northeast corner of Lake Aloha, traversing its length and displaying plenty of opportunities for camping among the many secluded alcoves above it—hidden from view and open to the stars.

Route Details

Start at the pleasant Echo Lake Chalet, and walk directly across the parking lot and over the metal causeway leading across Lower Echo Lake's dam and outlet. Watch for the hooks of anxious anglers as you

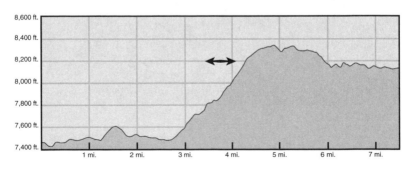

walk behind them; a polite "excuse me" is always understood to mean "keep your hooks out of my cheek." Follow the path to the right at the end of the bridge.

The trailhead is at the information kiosk for the TRT, where you can pick up a map for this section of the trail provided by the Tahoe Rim Trail Association. Climb the path northeast up to a clearing, past the point where your trail makes a sharp left, heading west. Walk east over to the edge of the clearing, and take in the magnificent vista of the South Lake Tahoe basin before beginning your route above Echo.

Because it's part of the PCT and TRT, it's no wonder the trail is in such excellent condition. Traverse the slightly rolling path roughly 100 feet above the shore, sometimes under cover of Jeffrey pines and sometimes on sunbaked granite. After a mile of westward travel, when Flagpole Peak is overhead, a brief switchback leads hikers away from a summer cabin access trail that veers off past a boulder. Now 200 feet above the lake, the trail squeezes beside the warm granite, and an excellent vista unfolds.

Under pleasant shade, the trail descends, intersects another cabin trail, and leads across granite at the northwest corner of Lower Echo Lake, where you have an excellent vista of Flagpole Peak over the lake. Round a small knob, and you can see the narrow channel that connects Upper and Lower Echo Lakes for the majority of the summer. Because Pacific Gas & Electric is able to draw down the top 12 feet of water in the lower of the two, this access for boats disappears late in the season. Until then, a water taxi is available on both lakes.

But this is a hike and not a boat ride, so continue your westward traverse along the smaller lake. First, descend across a lightly treed slope, then enter the trees about halfway down the lake. It's 0.6 mile to the water taxi dock from the knob where you first saw the channel. The sign for the water taxi, high in a tree, is easy to miss from either direction. There are three runoff streams just before you reach the trail to the dock. If you think you might want to take the boat ride on the way back, mark this spot. The fare is $12 per person, with a $36 minimum.

Climb at a steady pace as you leave the Echo lakes behind. Cross a runoff stream and continue west. In 0.4 mile, you will enter the Desolation Wilderness, a reminder to you that rangers check for both overnight and day-hike permits. Twenty yards on is a signed junction with a trail to Triangle Lake, leading on to Echo Peak. Lodgepole pines shade your trail another 0.3 mile as you continue ascending. The stream crossings are well engineered along here.

The uphill dirt-and-duff trail leaves the lodgepoles and crosses a small stone bridge to a spectacular lookout over both Echo lakes and down onto Tamarack, Cagwin, and Ralston Lakes, and across to Ralston Peak. Bypass the trail down to Tamarack Lake, and continue uphill at a steady rate—about 450 feet over the next 0.8 mile. Reach Haypress Meadows just after passing another trail junction leading easily across the sagebrush- and paintbrush-covered slope to Triangle Lake.

Your destination is to the west, across the north boundary of Haypress Meadows. The trail to Lake of the Woods crosses it 0.3 mile ahead in a lush copse of trees. As you hike, another trail heads to the same lake less than 1,000 feet farther on. You'll meet another pair of trails to the same location when you approach and pass Lakes Lucille and Margery, two small lakes below the trail to the north. Between them is a signed junction for a trail that veers left leading to the southeastern corner of Lake Aloha.

Your trail descends to intersect Aloha just as the tree cover ends and the granite trail begins. Poised in front of the Alps-like arêtes of Pyramid, Agassiz, and Price, Lake Aloha greets first-time visitors with a welcoming blast of reflected light. Almost aglow on any day, the shallow waters of this artificial lake glisten above the granite floor. Traverse the sandy or rocky trail beneath Cracked Crag, and watch for another faint trail about 0.5 mile from the last trail junction. There you can slip over the shallow ridge down to Lake LeConte and find solitude for your campsite.

Hike about 0.5 mile beyond a small peninsula of rock to reach the next trail junction—east to Heather Lake and west to Mosquito Pass and Clyde Lake. Take the westward trail, and begin looking for one of the many possible bivy sites located below the trail but still more than 200 feet from shore. Short hikes from camp will yield some huge vistas for those who choose to rest here beneath Jacks Peak.

Directions

From South Lake Tahoe, drive 4.8 miles south on US 50 to Meyers. Stay on US 50 past CA 89 for 5 more miles, then turn right onto Johnson Pass Road. This is a sharp right turn off of a long bend around Echo Summit, so here are some checkpoints: There is a Caltrans maintenance station at the tip of the bend (3.8 miles from Meyers). Your turn is a sharp right 1.2 miles ahead, just past the renovation-ready Little Norway.

From Placerville, drive 39.8 miles to Strawberry. Johnson Pass Road is on the left, 7.4 miles past Strawberry and 1.8 miles past Sierra-at-Tahoe ski resort. Follow the angled road as above.

Drive 0.6 mile along Johnson Pass Road to a left turn onto Echo Lakes Road, and stay left 0.9 mile, until you reach the large parking lot above the Echo Lakes Chalet. You can unload packs but not park down below in front of the chalet, but it's pretty easy to park up top and take the trail and steps leading from the north side of the lot down through the trees, behind the pit toilets, to the chalet.

Lake LeConte

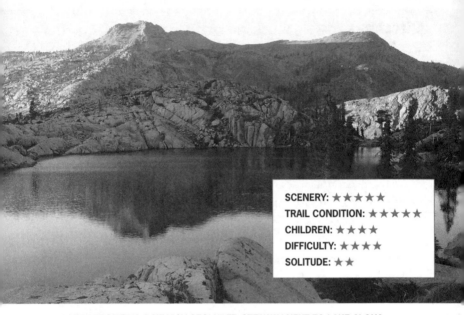

LAKE LECONTE IS A NEARLY SECLUDED GETAWAY NEXT TO LAKE ALOHA.

SCENERY: ★ ★ ★ ★ ★
TRAIL CONDITION: ★ ★ ★ ★ ★
CHILDREN: ★ ★ ★ ★
DIFFICULTY: ★ ★ ★ ★
SOLITUDE: ★ ★

GPS TRAILHEAD COORDINATES: N38° 50.125′ W120° 02.664′

DISTANCE & CONFIGURATION: 14.5-mile out-and-back

HIKING TIME: 8 hours (overnight)

OUTSTANDING FEATURES: Easy access to a dozen more stunning lakes is eclipsed by the dazzling display of granite presented by the Crystal Range; towering overhead are Pyramid and Ralston, Price and Jacks, Cracked Crag and Echo Peaks.

ELEVATION: 7,425′ at trailhead

ACCESS: Depends on snow; permits required for day hiking and overnight camping

MAPS: *Desolation Wilderness* (Wilderness Press)

FACILITIES: Pit toilet

COMMENTS: Bring sunglasses and sunscreen.

CONTACTS: Eldorado National Forest, Amador Ranger District, 209-295-4251, www.fs.usda.gov/eldorado; US Forest Service, Lake Tahoe Basin Management Unit, 530-543-2600, www.fs.usda.gov/ltbmu

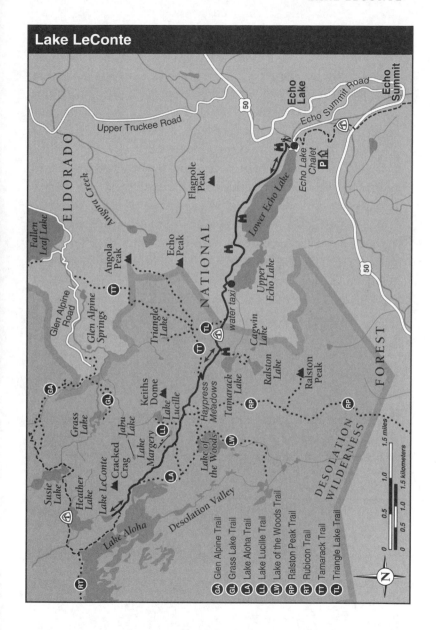

Lake LeConte

Overview

The trail to Lake Aloha presents no navigation challenges, although a compass and a map need to be among your essentials. Although many side trails to lakes intersect your route, this is part of both the Pacific Crest Trail (PCT) and Tahoe Rim Trail (TRT), so the signage is fresh, accurate, and present at (nearly) every junction.

The PCT traverses steadily northwest past a half-dozen small, medium, and large lakes before steering to this diminutive lake. There are other ones this size and smaller to be enjoyed, so your route visits Jabu Lake on the way in and Lakes Margery and Lucille on the way out.

The Desolation Wilderness is one of the most visited back-country areas in California. Because of its proximity to the Bay Area and Sacramento and its easily accessible trailheads, this entry to the Desolation Wilderness is always highly trafficked, and so there are daily quotas for overnight camping, which can fill five months in advance for weekends. Day hikers are asked to register at the trail-head or at a US Forest Service visitor center at no charge; overnight campers must pay to secure a permit. A good place to do that online is here: tinyurl.com/dwovernightcamping.

Route Details

Start at the pleasant Echo Lake Chalet, and walk over the concrete dam and the metal causeway across Lower Echo Lake's outlet. Pausing

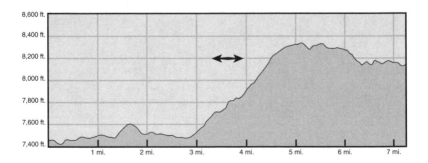

for photos here is a ritual, but be sure to keep out of the way of spinning lures.

The trail begins at the TRT information kiosk, where the Tahoe Rim Trail Association provides section maps. At the top of this brief climb, your trail makes a sharp left, heading west. There's another great vista, however, just across the clearing to the northeast. Take in this magnificent vista of the South Lake Tahoe basin before beginning your route above Echo.

Traverse the slightly rolling path roughly 100 feet above the shore, sometimes under cover of Jeffrey pines and sometimes on sunbaked granite. After a mile of westward travel, when Flagpole Peak is overhead, a brief switchback leads hikers away from a summer cabin access trail that veers off past a boulder. Now 200 feet above the lake, the trail squeezes beside the warm granite, and an excellent vista unfolds.

Descend under some pleasant shade and across granite at the northwest corner of Lower Echo Lake, where you have an excellent vista of Flagpole Peak. Round a small knob, and you can see the narrow channel that connects Upper and Lower Echo Lakes for the majority of the summer. Because Pacific Gas & Electric is able to draw down the top 12 feet of water in the lower of the two, this access for boats disappears late in the season in normal snowfall years. Until this level drops, a water taxi is available on both lakes.

But this is a hike and not a boat ride, so continue your westward traverse along the smaller lake. First, descend across a lightly treed slope, then enter the trees about halfway down the lake. It's 0.6 mile to the water taxi dock from the knob where you first saw the channel. The sign for the water taxi, high in a tree, is easy to miss from either direction. There are three runoff streams just before you reach the trail to the dock. If you think you might want to take the boat ride on the way back, mark this spot. The fare is $12 per person, with a $36 minimum.

Climb at a steady pace as you leave the Echo lakes behind. Cross a runoff stream and continue west. In 0.4 mile, you enter the

Desolation Wilderness, a reminder to you that rangers check for both overnight and day-hike permits. Twenty yards on is a signed junction with a trail to Triangle Lake, leading on to Echo Peak. Lodgepole pines shade your trail for another 0.3 mile as you continue ascending. The stream crossings are well engineered along here.

The uphill dirt-and-duff trail leaves the lodgepoles and crosses a small stone bridge to a spectacular lookout over both Echo lakes and down onto Tamarack, Cagwin, and Ralston Lakes, and across to Ralston Peak. Bypass the trail down to Tamarack Lake, and continue uphill at a steady rate—about 450 feet over the next 0.8 mile. You will reach Haypress Meadows just after passing another trail junction leading easily across the sagebrush- and paintbrush-covered slope to Triangle Lake.

Your destination is to the west, across the north boundary of Haypress Meadows. The trail to Lake of the Woods crosses it 0.3 mile ahead in a lush copse of trees. As you hike, another trail heads to the same lake less than 1,000 feet farther on. You'll meet another pair of trails to the same location when you approach and pass Lakes Lucille and Margery. These two small lakes are below the trail to the north. Between them is a signed junction for a trail that veers off to the left, leading to the southeastern corner of Lake Aloha. On the way in, you can bypass all of these trails and remain on the PCT.

However, if you want to go where no other hikers will be enjoying the vista, I suggest a 0.5-mile diversion north to Jabu Lake. Soon after the second trail marker for Lucille and Margery, turn right, uphill to the north-northwest, on the shallow talus-and-gravel slope. Jabu, named for Echo local Jack Butler, is about 200 feet to the north. A night on the western margin of this tiny pond is sheltered, quiet, and star-soaked. Sunset views over Aloha include the Crystal Range and a dawn vista of Fallen Leaf Lake and Mount Tallac.

Descend to intersect the PCT at Aloha just as the tree cover ends and the granite trail begins. Poised in front of the Alps-like arêtes of Pyramid, Agassiz, and Price, Lake Aloha greets first-time visitors with a welcoming blast of reflected light. Traverse the sandy

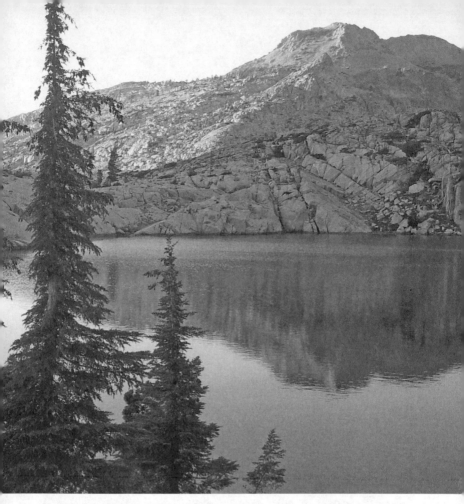

MOUNTAIN HEMLOCK ON THE EASTERN SHORE OF LAKE LeCONTE

or rocky trail, watching for another faint trail about 0.5 mile from the last trail junction. There you can slip down below the trail to find a bivy spot at Lake LeConte.

Named after John LeConte, the noted geologist and physician famous for the diagnosis "you've got rocks in your head," Lake LeConte has limited views as it sits in a rock-rimmed bowl—usually unseen by trail traffic. The warm water of this small lake makes summer afternoon dips quite pleasant. Nice bivy sites are most easily found at the south end of the lake, where some firs and scattered pines add texture to the granite.

If you're feeling well rested and want just a bit more hiking, on the way out you can easily detour to the east on a 0.5-mile forested, downhill trail leading past Margery and on to some nice picnic spots near Lucille. Take a left at the first signed junction after departing Aloha's shore. Your trail is shaded on this entire detour and continues on the southeast side of the creek. Skirt the lake about 200 feet and then, uphill about the same distance, back to the PCT but more directly south.

From your intersection with the PCT, you'll turn left and be back at the chalet in exactly 5 miles.

Directions

From South Lake Tahoe, drive 4.8 miles south on US 50 to Meyers. Stay on US 50 past CA 89 for 5 more miles, then turn right onto Johnson Pass Road. This is a sharp right turn off of a long bend around Echo Summit, so here are some checkpoints: There is a Caltrans maintenance station at the tip of the bend (3.8 miles from Meyers). Your turn is a sharp right 1.2 miles ahead, just past the renovation-ready Little Norway.

From Placerville, drive 39.8 miles to Strawberry. Johnson Pass Road is on the left, 7.4 miles past Strawberry and 1.8 miles past Sierra-at-Tahoe ski resort. Follow the angled road as above.

Drive 0.6 mile along Johnson Pass Road to a left turn onto Echo Lakes Road; stay left 0.9 mile, until you reach the large parking lot above the Echo Lakes Chalet. You can unload packs but not park down below in front of the chalet, but it's pretty easy to park up top and take the trail and steps leading from the north side of the lot down through the trees, behind the pit toilets, to the chalet.

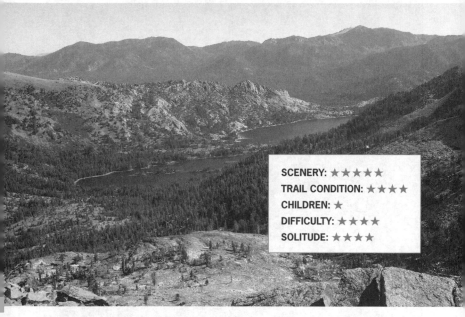

SCENERY: ★ ★ ★ ★ ★
TRAIL CONDITION: ★ ★ ★ ★
CHILDREN: ★
DIFFICULTY: ★ ★ ★ ★
SOLITUDE: ★ ★ ★ ★

THE ECHO LAKES ARE NESTLED BELOW RALSTON PEAK AND ABOVE TAHOE.

GPS TRAILHEAD COORDINATES: N38° 48.291′ W120° 06.936′

DISTANCE & CONFIGURATION: 7.2–7.6-mile balloon loop

HIKING TIME: 6.5 hours

OUTSTANDING FEATURES: Flower-filled meadows brighten the fir- and hemlock-adorned slopes. Knockout vistas include Pyramid Peak; Mount Tallac; and the lakes of Desolation Valley, including Aloha and Echo with several others in between. You also have a peek at distant Fallen Leaf Lake and Lake Tahoe.

ELEVATION: 6,506′ at trailhead

ACCESS: Depends on snow; permits required for day hiking and overnight camping

MAPS: *Desolation Wilderness* (Wilderness Press)

FACILITIES: None

COMMENTS: Carry plenty of water.

CONTACTS: Eldorado National Forest, Amador Ranger District, 209-295-4251, www.fs.usda.gov/eldorado; US Forest Service, Lake Tahoe Basin Management Unit, 530-543-2600, www.fs.usda.gov/ltbmu

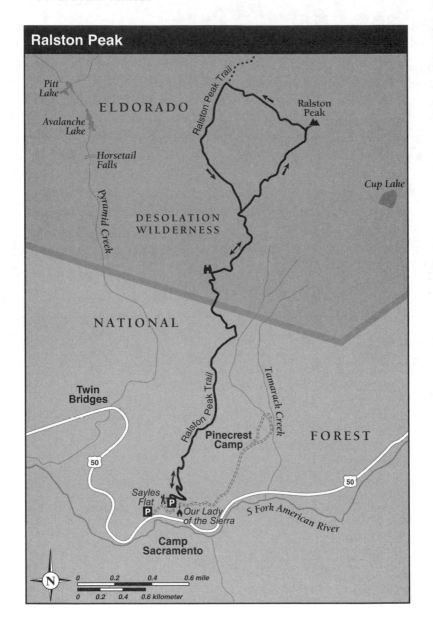

Ralston Peak

Pitt Lake

Avalanche Lake

ELDORADO

Ralston Peak Trail

Ralston Peak

Horsetail Falls

Cup Lake

Pyramid Creek

DESOLATION WILDERNESS

NATIONAL

Twin Bridges

Ralston Peak Trail

Tamarack Creek

Pinecrest Camp

FOREST

50

50

Sayles Flat

P

P

Our Lady of the Sierra

S Fork American River

Camp Sacramento

N

| 0 | 0.2 | 0.4 | 0.6 mile |

| 0 | 0.2 | 0.4 | 0.6 kilometer |

Overview

Incredible views of a dozen glacial lakes and prominent peaks from a vista point 1,100 feet above Desolation Valley are yours to enjoy as you begin ascending the lateral moraine forming Pyramid Creek's canyon. The trail climbs at a consistent rate for the first third of the hike then tests your lungs and legs for just over a mile before resuming a more reasonable slope to the summit.

Route Details

Once at the trailhead, take time to fill out a Desolation Wilderness day-hike permit and attach it to your pack. Day permits are free; overnight campers must pay to secure a permit. A good place to do that online is here: tinyurl.com/dwovernightcamping.

A few switchbacks send you traversing through the Jeffrey pines and white firs that shade you at the outset on the flank of this ice-carved chunk of rock. A beautiful vista point lies less than 0.3 mile from the trailhead. As you stand in this open, sandy spot, Pyramid Creek's canyon spreads out in front of you like a gaping tear in the mountain.

You will have traversed northeast 1.1 miles before some serious switchbacks hand you about 1,250 feet of elevation gain in the next 1.1 miles. The Desolation Wilderness boundary sign, about 1.6 miles along, will be a reminder that you need a wilderness permit.

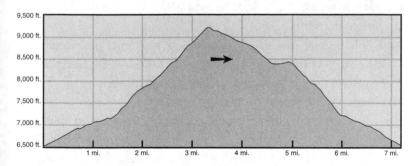

From this point, about 950 feet above the trailhead, you can glimpse the Sierra-at-Tahoe ski runs to the south.

After another 300 feet of elevation gain, your way will appear to be blocked by an unnecessarily large boulder, which you will just have to clamber over to continue on this well-defined, steep, sandy trail. More large boulders sitting 1.5 miles from the trailhead offer a nice location for a quick break, where you can pretend to take pictures while you catch your breath.

The trail will occasionally be tightly bordered by huckleberry oak, manzanita, bush chinquapin, and buckbrush ceanothus. And magnificent vistas. Turn away from your wall-to-wall view of Pyramid Peak and traverse east across the south-facing slope. In about 300 feet, you'll step across a stagnant spring seeping water from beneath a boulder. In another 300 feet, your path turns northeast again.

Continue climbing another 200 feet to a pleasant south-facing meadow adorned with pinemat manzanita and buckwheat. Turn northwest and climb another 250 feet to crest a small ridge. Here, your trail divides, with one option turning right (northeast) or continuing directly ahead (northwest). To the right is an unofficial trail to the summit that has been improved because of its popularity.

The trail to the northeast is shorter by almost 1 mile, but its average grade is twice as steep as the northwest route. They are both spectacular, and I will describe the *ascent* of them both. The mapped route takes this path up and the longer path down. I will begin with the path to the right.

This is really steep. Not Pyramid Peak steep, but really steep nonetheless. And the beginning of it is the easy part. So, with the gentle path to the northwest fading in the distance, your route will be very clear as you trudge 0.75 mile uphill across the open slope decorated with pine and hemlock. The switchbacks are sometimes tight as the sandy trail maneuvers between the boulders and among the trees.

For entertainment during this leg workout, you may notice some of the approximately 6,107 ducks—rock trail markers—that have been erected to guide you safely to the summit. With plenty of

ducks and dozens of footprints in the sand, your navigation requirements on this trail are fairly minimal. But it's fun to have a map
along, if for no other reason than to identify the peaks and lakes that
surround you. They are especially visible on this approach. As you
near the summit, a large cairn and, unbelievably, more ducks stand in
your way—or guide you to the top. Actually, any route to the summit
here is attainable. Just use good balance and move uphill.

If you choose the longer path, this 1,500-foot traverse to the
northwest begins with a shallow descent from the ridgecrest. About
the time you reach a meadow fed by a seasonal stream, your route
will turn north. Lupine, corn lily, Indian paintbrush, asters, and
meadow penstemon color this south-sloping patch where flickers and
woodpeckers pound at the snags and yellow-rumped warblers chase
through the pine.

Your uphill trail leads less than 0.5 mile to the junction with
the trail to the summit. You may share your path with a seasonal
runoff stream along here. The Western white pines' pendant cones,
heavy with sap, glisten in the sun as you make your way through
them and mountain hemlock to the junction marked by a modest
cairn. A longer hike with a bit less elevation gain leads to this point
from the Echo lakes via Haypress Meadows.

Turn east-southeast at this junction for a pleasant half-mile
hike through scattered Western hemlock. The whistles you hear from
the rock field to the north come from the several marmots whose territory you are entering. Watch your trail closely and look back to see
where you're coming from (an aim point) so that you don't take an
incorrect heading on your return.

The sandy trail leads to the base of the rockfall, just 100 feet
below the summit. A brief climb up this talus cap will reward you
with 360-degree views—from Lake Tahoe in the distance to Lakes
Ralston, Cagwin, and Tamarack beneath you. Your vista includes
Lovers Leap, Pyramid Peak, Jacks and Dicks Peaks, Cracked Crag
and Mount Tallac, and distant Freel Peak. The views of Lake of the
Woods, Lake Aloha, and Echo Lakes are spectacular.

If you're not too busy battling the butterflies on the summit, you may notice the shaggy hawkweed—a fuzzy, yellow-flowered plant glistening in the sun. You'll probably also see several golden-mantled ground squirrels darting around looking for handouts. Do them a favor and don't feed them. Before heading down, look for your aim point so you don't inadvertently head too far downhill to the north.

Directions

The trailhead parking lot in Sayles Flat is on the left side of US 50, just 2.5 miles east of Strawberry (40 miles east of Placerville). Watch for signs for Camp Sacramento.

If coming from the east, the trailhead is on the right past Echo Summit, exactly 2.75 miles west of the Sierra-at-Tahoe ski area (which is 10.7 miles west of South Lake Tahoe).

The generous parking lot along the broad shoulder of the highway is signed for Ralston Peak and the Our Lady of the Sierra chapel. You can park here or drive about 200 yards up the dirt road, where there is room for four cars to park at the trailhead to the left of the tiny church.

Pyramid Peak

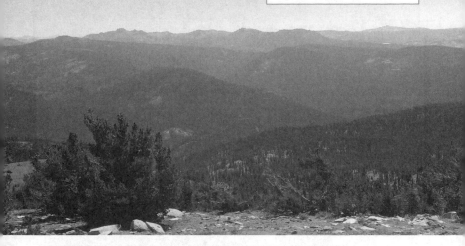

LOOKING SOUTH PAST SIERRA-AT-TAHOE SKI AREA TO THE NIPPLE.

SCENERY: ★ ★ ★ ★ ★	
TRAIL CONDITION: ★ ★ ★ ★	
CHILDREN: ★	
DIFFICULTY: ★ ★ ★ ★ ★	
SOLITUDE: ★ ★ ★ ★	

GPS TRAILHEAD COORDINATES: N38° 48.501′ W120° 08.156′

DISTANCE & CONFIGURATION: 7.7-mile out-and-back

HIKING TIME: 8 hours

OUTSTANDING FEATURES: Panoramic vista of the Crystal Range and the Desolation Wilderness; views from Lake Tahoe to Loon Lake, including Lake Aloha, Echo Lakes, and Fallen Leaf Lake; and clear views to the south, including Elephants Back, Round Top, Thimble Peak, and The Nipple

ELEVATION: 6,033′ at trailhead

ACCESS: Year-round

MAPS: *Desolation Wilderness* (Wilderness Press)

FACILITIES: None

COMMENTS: Be sure to carry plenty of water.

CONTACT: Eldorado National Forest, Amador Ranger District, 209-295-4251, www.fs.usda.gov/eldorado

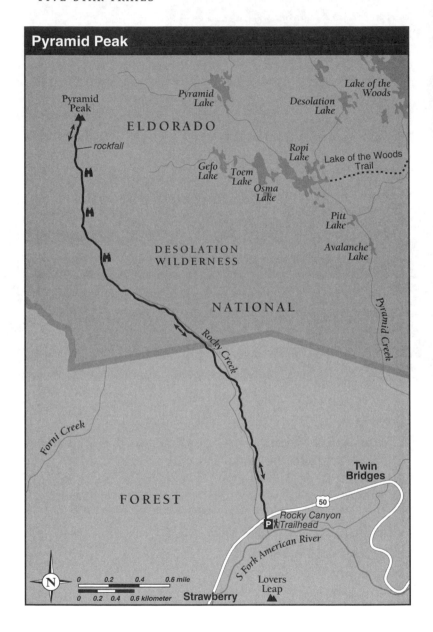

Pyramid Peak

Pyramid
Peak

rockfall

ELDORADO

Pyramid
Lake

Lake of the
Woods

Desolation
Lake

Ropi
Lake

Lake of the Woods
Trail

Gefo
Lake

Toem
Lake

Osma
Lake

Pitt
Lake

DESOLATION
WILDERNESS

Avalanche
Lake

NATIONAL

Pyramid Creek

Rocky Creek

Forni Creek

Twin
Bridges

FOREST

50

Rocky Canyon
Trailhead

S Fork American River

Lovers
Leap

N

| 0 | 0.2 | 0.4 | 0.6 mile |

| 0 | 0.2 | 0.4 | 0.6 kilometer |

Strawberry

Overview

Four thousand feet of elevation gain—straight up—had better have an incredibly redeeming quality besides aerobic exercise, and Pyramid Peak via Rocky Canyon dishes it up for hearty hikers only. The views alone are worth the hike up this triangle of granite talus. But the solitude, the adventure, and even the workout will leave you with a feeling of well-being and a sense of accomplishment. This is perhaps the hardest hike in the book.

Route Details

Hikers have more than a few ways to hike to Pyramid Peak, but the route up Rocky Canyon is definitely the most strenuous. And for every small, strained, uphill step you take, there will be a surprising reward along the trail. Your reward at the top may be more brilliant than you anticipated.

You won't find the trail up Rocky Canyon marked on current maps; nor is it marked at the trailhead. Before crossing to the north side of the road, you should be able to spot one of the two faint trails that ascend the steep bank on large rocks in the dirt. Traffic is very close here, so choose your spot carefully. The trails are almost opposite the 43-mile milestone, which is 500 feet to the east.

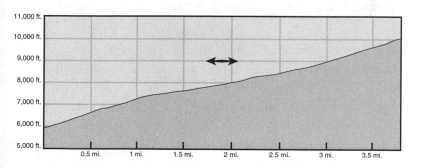

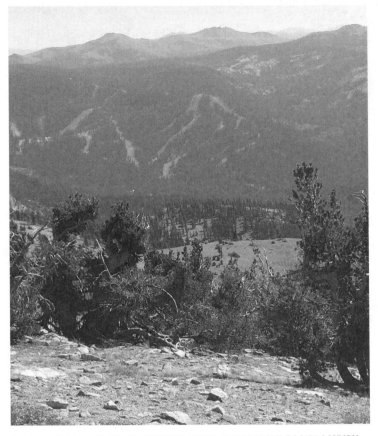

SKI SLOPES AS SEEN FROM PYRAMID'S SOUTH FLANK ABOVE ROCKY CANYON

Once atop the bank, you will see a large log across the trail. Maneuver around the log and you'll spot the trail. Continue uphill another 100 vertical feet and avoid a false trail to the left. Instead, make sure to go right and stay away from the creek. You'll come close to the stream and eventually cross it, but not for a little while. If you're catching your breath after another 125 vertical feet, turn around and take a fresh look at Lovers Leap. From this vantage point, you can clearly see the small dome in front of what looks like a miniature version of Yosemite's famous monolith, Half Dome.

Another 100 vertical feet brings you to yet another speed bump that looks like it used to be an incense cedar. While you are on this pleasant part of the dirt-and-duff trail, you're shaded by Jeffrey pine, white fir, and incense cedar. Manzanita crowds the trail frequently in this forested section. Avoid another false trail to the left and continue climbing. At about 6,350 feet, you get your first clear glimpse of Rocky Creek, although there is no way to reach it from this point.

Keep climbing on the stream's east side, seemingly vertical at times, through the mixed conifer forest. As if you were going too fast, another speed bump has been placed in your trail—a fir that has been trodden upon so much it has the feel of balsa wood.

Your short switchbacks on this dirt-and-duff trail lead through an area littered with deadfall right around the 7,000-foot contour. Intermittently, the trail turns to sand and rock or scree. As it comes a bit closer to the stream, the only bird you may hear is a Steller's jay, although you'll find woodpeckers and grouse slightly higher.

If you're here early in the season, you'll find the trail to be a muddy stream nearly everywhere. All of that meltwater carries the seeds that flow down across the trail, leaving behind a display of lupine, aster, and Indian paintbrush alongside snow plant and pinedrops. Within sound of the creek, willows and flowers become quite dense along the sandy trail. A gentle breeze along here will shake the leaves of this grove of aspens.

The crossing at Rocky Creek, about elevation 7,350, is an easy one brightened by mountain bluebells, red and yellow columbine, dense ferns, and paintbrush.

Once on the west side of the stream, you will ascend gradually through Jeffrey and lodgepole pines along a huge granite outcrop. Skirt the flank of this outcrop, bouncing between the stream on the right and the outcrop on the left. Duck beneath a fallen lodgepole, and then walk around the prone fir. Then resume your climbing among the lupine and pinemat manzanita. Plenty of colorful flowers will greet you when you pass through the next small, sloping meadow.

Right around 8,000 feet in elevation, you will have 250 vertical feet of short, steep, almost unfair trail that mimics a wavy sliding board with sand. But of all things, you'll find a nearly flat spot surrounded by willows, asters, corn lilies, and cobalt-blue sky. The little knoll to the left appears as if it would support at least one tent beneath the towering fir. You may see a Western white pine with a hollow space at its base, which on closer examination reveals a boulder that the tree swallowed as it grew.

Just as you pass the last little meadow, where two or three meltwater streams converge and where another bivy site could be located to the west, you will first spy your destination. Silhouetted against a cloudless sky, Pyramid Peak strikes an imposing figure to a tired hiker at this vantage point of 8,500 feet. Make your way across the jumbled maze of broken rock, where several ducks have been accurately laid out to mark the trail.

A set of absolutely brutal switchbacks send you up the pinkish granite to the top of this steep rock wall. When you reach the top of that winding course, your trail will be clear—and vertical—in front of you, and although the trail is very narrow, it's quite distinct. The path traverses to the east side of the slope and then continues on some ridiculously sadistic switchbacks, brightened only by the mountain heather growing trailside that guides you straight uphill directly toward the peak.

While you're busy hydrating, turn to the south to get a good view of the Sierra-at-Tahoe Ski Resort beneath you as well as some distant views of some of the peaks in the Mokelumne Wilderness: Elephants Back, Round Top, Thimble Peak, and The Nipple.

By 9,500 feet, your well-marked trail switches back and forth through scattered and crippled pines that provide no shade or cover from the sun overhead. Just after another turn, Pyramid's talus slope looms up in front of you. You have only 450 vertical feet until the summit, where some well-constructed circular windbreaks can accommodate lots of hiking companions.

The line in front of you is fairly easy and about as good as it gets across the entire south face. This is very easy Class 3 hiking. You may encounter some points where you will need to use your hands to maintain balance on these large granite boulders. Continue straight up to the summit, or work your way to the west as you ascend. Pay attention to avoid the steep ascent on the east face, and you'll be at the top rather quickly.

While you're climbing up you may see a marmot or two. I was greeted at the summit by thousands and thousands of California tortoiseshell butterflies that, once disturbed, flowed from the summit down the path I had ascended. Thirty minutes later, at the base of the rockfall, the flying orange flowers persisted in their downhill deluge.

Linger at the summit to take pictures of this magnificent range that the glaciers sculpted and of the lakes they left behind. Keep a close eye on changes in the weather—summer thunderstorms are dangerous and can be counted on by 3 p.m. in the Tahoe area.

Directions

This informal trailhead is located on the north shoulder of US 50, halfway between Twin Bridges and Strawberry. A pullout with parking room for six or seven cars sits precisely beneath a programmable highway information sign, 43 miles east of Placerville on the south side of the road. The sign's silver control box sits at the west end of the pullout.

From your parking spot on the south side, you're about 500 feet west of the 43-mile milestone. Walk about 375 feet east along the highway, and locate one of the two faint trails that lead up the embankment on the opposite side of the road. The trail leads up to a fallen log across the obvious trail. At the log, the trail is quite visible and leads straight uphill.

This is a dangerous crossing because the fast-traveling traffic has little time to react. Look twice.

Half Moon, Alta Morris, and Gilmore Lakes

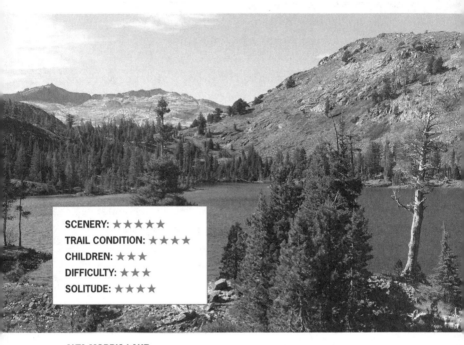

SCENERY: ★ ★ ★ ★ ★
TRAIL CONDITION: ★ ★ ★ ★
CHILDREN: ★ ★ ★
DIFFICULTY: ★ ★ ★
SOLITUDE: ★ ★ ★ ★

ALTA MORRIS LAKE

GPS TRAILHEAD COORDINATES: N38° 52.637′ W120° 04.846′

DISTANCE & CONFIGURATION: 13.3-mile out-and-back with spur and lake loop

HIKING TIME: 5 hours

OUTSTANDING FEATURES: Visit three backcountry lakes for camping or wildflower photography. Both reports and lies about fish abound. You'll be treated to spectacular views of the 1,300-foot-tall lithic palisades of the largest cirque in the Desolation Wilderness.

ELEVATION: 6,515′ at trailhead

ACCESS: Depends on snow; permits required for day hiking and overnight camping

MAPS: *Desolation Wilderness* (Wilderness Press)

FACILITIES: Pit toilet

CONTACT: US Forest Service, Taylor Creek Visitor Center, 530-543-2674, tinyurl.com/taylorcreekvisitorcenter

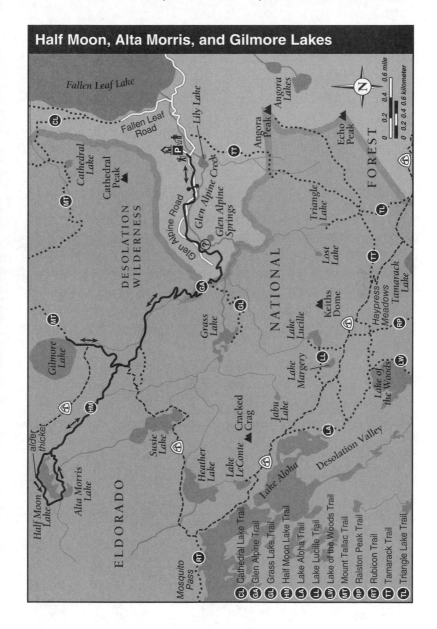

Half Moon, Alta Morris, and Gilmore Lakes

Fallen Leaf Lake

Lily Lake

Angora Lakes

Angora Peak

Echo Peak

N

0.6 mile
0.4
0.2
0
0 0.2 0.4 0.6 kilometer

Fallen Leaf Road

FOREST

Cathedral Lake

Cathedral Peak

Glen Alpine Creek

Glen Alpine Springs

Triangle Lake

DESOLATION WILDERNESS

Glen Alpine Road

Grass Lake

Lost Lake

Keiths Dome

Haypress Meadows

Tamarack Lake

Gilmore Lake

Lake Lucille

NATIONAL

alder thicket

Half Moon Lake

Alta Morris Lake

Susie Lake

Heather Lake

Lake LeConte

Cracked Crag

Jabu Lake

Lake Margery

Lake of the Woods

Desolation Valley

ELDORADO

Lake Aloha

Mosquito Pass

Cathedral Lake Trail
Glen Alpine Trail
Grass Lake Trail
Half Moon Lake Trail
Lake Aloha Trail
Lake Lucille Trail
Lake of the Woods Trail
Mount Tallac Trail
Ralston Peak Trail
Rubicon Trail
Tamarack Trail
Triangle Lake Trail

CL GA GL HM LA LL LW MT RP RT TT TL

Overview

The trail follows Glen Alpine Creek past its namesake spring and resort before making a brief ascent to its source at Gilmore Lake via the Pacific Crest Trail (PCT). The cirque surrounding circular Gilmore certainly is impressive and picturesque, but the crowds that stop here on weekends can be avoided by descending to a massive, deep cirque cradling tiny Alta Morris and aptly named Half Moon Lakes. There, campsites and solitude are generous offerings.

Route Details

Depart the trailhead and skirt the beaver-inhabited Lily Lake on a forest road surfaced with baseball-sized scree. Follow the road and the trail signs that lead past cabins and waterfalls as described in Hike 23, Glen Alpine Loop. Pass the resort and springs, where an information kiosk will fill you in on the area's history. The cool, dim light under the pines will not last much longer, as your exposed trail begins at the marker just ahead for Grass Lake and Susie Lake.

Climb steadily south and then turn west for the Desolation Wilderness, which you enter 1.75 miles from the trailhead. (Did you remember to get a permit?) Fill up your water bottles 0.4 mile ahead, just prior to a shaded flat where there's a marker indicating Grass Lake to the left and Susie Lake and Mount Tallac, your trail, on ahead. Climb slightly through tree cover along the creek's border up to some easy switchbacks that carry you up the face of this slope. A

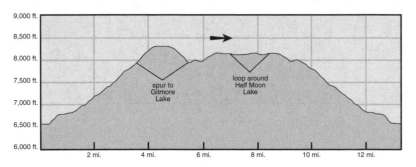

pleasant forest shades you for about 0.5 mile beginning at about 2.5 miles along. After a brief taste of near-horizontal terrain among these lodgepole pines, continue an easy uphill on a manzanita-lined trail. Vistas open up on the switchbacks, so have your camera available.

Cross another shaded stream just before the trail turns to the northwest. An interesting crossing of Glen Alpine Creek lies 0.5 mile ahead where, early in the season, the rushing water requires careful consideration before taking a step. After midseason, the stream disappears from 100 feet upstream to 100 feet downstream, leaving a simple and dry crossing. Just ahead is a trail marker for a three-way junction; the trail to Susie and Aloha Lakes heads left, and your track to the right leads to Dicks Pass.

Take off to the northwest on the gravel trail and stairs heading toward the junction with the PCT 0.25 mile ahead. A link to the PCT leads left to Echo Lakes while you head right to Gilmore Lake. Twenty-five feet up the trail is another junction offering a path to Half Moon and Alta Morris Lakes (which you'll take later) to the left. The signed link on the PCT to Lake Aloha requires a sharp left partially hidden behind the large boulder. And the trail to Gilmore is to the right.

Less than 0.75 mile away, and only slightly uphill, Gilmore Lake (of Glen Alpine Resort fame) squats below a heavily carved cirque. The PCT departs for Dicks Pass, off to the west about 300 yards before reaching this lake. Gilmore's shores are tree-splattered on the south and east, where a few social trails lead to some highly impacted campsites that are too close to the shore. To the west and north, the waters are contained by steep, rocky slopes that would send tents sliding into the shallow water.

Cross the nascent Glen Alpine Creek to find some good bivy sites and the trail to Mount Tallac. If camping here, a trip up to Tallac is well worth it. Follow the trail uphill from the marker that stands 150 feet northeast of the dam. Hike up to another marker below the summit. For directions from here, turn to the next hike, Mount Tallac (page 170).

Including the trail that you retrace, you will reach Half Moon Lake in about 2 miles. Return to the intersection with the Glen Alpine Trail, and turn sharply right, heading uphill slightly on broken rock. Your destination is roughly 1 mile ahead. With the massive wall of the cirque to the right, your vistas are limited to southerly views as you ascend and descend this broken rock. Blazes persist in old trees and remain accurate for navigating along here. Pass by a few seasonal puddles and a small, boggy meadow decorated with mountain alder, corn lily, paintbrush, larkspur, and Sierra gentian.

The trail, mostly lined by mountain heather and pussytoes, continues traversing northwest beneath a slope filled with a combination of pinemat manzanita, lupine, paintbrush, aster, and chinquapin.

The ridge to the northeast separates this cirque from Gilmore's, and it has dropped a huge load of rock from its flanks. Sagebrush and fireweed add color to the hillside as you pass a large puddle south of the trail.

Meander along the creek a bit more, and then climb over a small bump and down to a tiny pond fed by a runoff stream with a copse of junipers and lodgepole pines on its north side.

You can descend to Half Moon and circumnavigate it via your trail. While it does become overgrown and boggy in places on the north side of the lake, the wildflowers here below Dicks Peak are thick late into the season. You can continue around to Alta Morris Lake this way, but it becomes very wet for a few hundred feet. A better plan, if you want to bivy near Alta Morris (and you should), is to head crosscountry after the tiny pond before initially descending to Half Moon.

To do that, head west over the crumbling, undulating terrain. The granite above the south shore of Half Moon Lake also has a couple of bivy sites on either side of its outlet stream. From Half Moon's shore, trend southwest, winding through variable ponds for 1,000 feet. Stay between Alta Morris's outlet and a small pond that receives the lake's cascade. Walk above the meltwater puddles toward the tiny land bridge. Acceptable bivy sites are located on the bench above Alta Morris, where the moon will light up the night reflected off this massive granite amphitheater. Dicks Peak, as well as the Dicks Pass and Lake, was named in memory of Captain Richard Barter, "the hermit of Emerald Bay" who drowned there in 1875.

Directions

Fallen Leaf Lake Road is located off CA 89, 3.1 miles north of South Lake Tahoe and 24.1 miles south of Tahoe City. Turn from the highway onto Fallen Leaf Lake Road and, in 0.1 mile, take the left fork. Drive 4.7 miles along the narrow and winding road circumnavigating Fallen Leaf Lake, past Tahoe Mountain Road, to the marina at the junction of Fallen Leaf Lake Road and Glen Alpine Road. Bear left on Glen Alpine Road, and follow it 0.6 mile to the trailhead parking lot. This road may be closed yearly from November to April.

The lot is equipped with pit toilets, trash receptacles, and plenty of parking. The trailhead kiosk holds a supply of free day-hike permits, which are required for travel in the Desolation Wilderness. Overnight stays require a paid camping permit, which can be secured locally at the Taylor Creek Visitor Center, 150 yards to the west of Fallen Leaf Lake Road on CA 89, or online at tinyurl.com/dwovernightcamping.

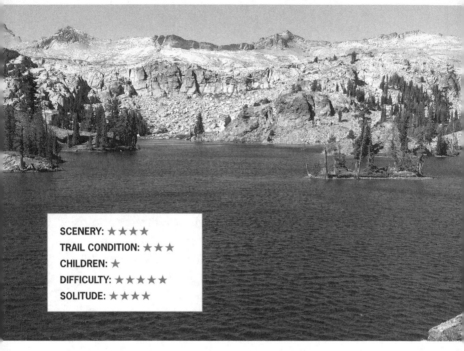

HEATHER LAKE WITH THE CRYSTAL RANGE IN THE DISTANCE

SCENERY: ★ ★ ★
TRAIL CONDITION: ★ ★ ★
CHILDREN: ★
DIFFICULTY: ★ ★ ★ ★ ★
SOLITUDE: ★ ★ ★

GPS TRAILHEAD COORDINATES: N38° 52.637′ W120° 04.846′

DISTANCE & CONFIGURATION: 13.4-mile loop

HIKING TIME: 8–9 hours

OUTSTANDING FEATURES: Lakes, peaks, and vistas are in plentiful supply as you hike through thick forest and glaciated terrain. Name your pleasure: waterfalls, cascades, beaver ponds, meadows, polished granite, fragrant wildflowers, or trees. This is one of my favorites because of its varied terrain and vegetation.

ELEVATION: 6,629′ at trailhead

ACCESS: Depends on snow; permits required for day hiking and overnight camping

MAPS: *Desolation Wilderness* (Wilderness Press)

FACILITIES: Pit toilet

CONTACT: US Forest Service, Taylor Creek Visitor Center, 530-543-2674, tinyurl.com/taylorcreekvisitorcenter

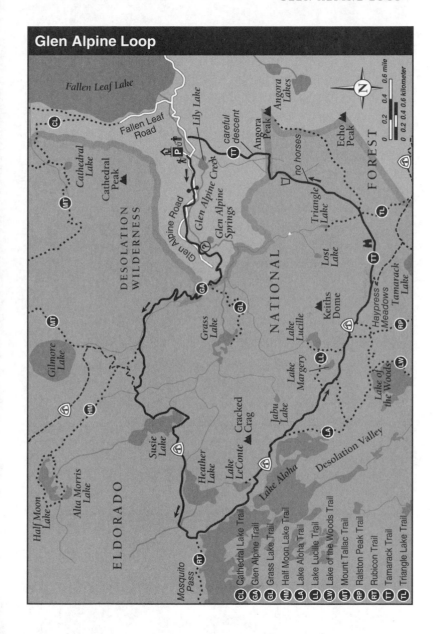

Glen Alpine Loop

Fallen Leaf Lake

Lily Lake

careful descent

Angora Lakes

Angora Peak

Echo Peak

FOREST

0   0.2   0.4   0.6 mile
0   0.2 0.4 0.6 kilometer

Fallen Leaf Road

no horses

Cathedral Lake

Cathedral Peak

Glen Alpine Creek

Glen Alpine Springs

Triangle Lake

DESOLATION WILDERNESS

Glen Alpine Road

Lost Lake

Tamarack Lake

NATIONAL

Grass Lake

Keiths Dome

Haypress Meadows

Gilmore Lake

Lake Lucille

Lake Margery

Lake of the Woods

Jabu Lake

Cracked Crag

Lake LeConte

Half Moon Lake

Alta Morris Lake

Susie Lake

Heather Lake

Lake Aloha

Desolation Valley

ELDORADO

Mosquito Pass

CL Cathedral Lake Trail
GA Glen Alpine Trail
GL Grass Lake Trail
HM Half Moon Lake Trail
JL Lake Aloha Trail
LL Lake Lucille Trail
LW Lake of the Woods Trail
MT Mount Tallac Trail
RP Ralston Peak Trail
RT Rubicon Trail
TT Tamarack Trail
TL Triangle Lake Trail

Overview

Ready yourself for varied terrain as you climb away from your trail-head, situated between Angora and Cathedral Peaks. Pass historic Glen Alpine Springs Resort while ascending its namesake creek to the west. Linger at lightly treed Susie Lake, where Jacks and Dicks Peaks loom in the background. Climb to the outlet stream of rockbound Heather Lake's azure waters, brightened by the polished snow-clad Crystal Range. Briefly ascend to Lake Aloha, where your viewfinder will be full of Pyramid, Agassiz, and Price looming overhead. Mosey along Aloha's shore over granite, and then take an uphill path away from Lake of the Woods, heading toward Haypress Meadows. Forgo the easy trails down to Echo, and view a trio of lakes—Ralston, Cagwin, and Tamarack—from your high route toward Triangle Lake. Return to Lily Lake by descending the steep Tamarack Trail, which is laden with vistas of Tahoe and Fallen Leaf Lakes.

Route Details

Be certain to pick up a permit from the kiosk located adjacent to the trailhead, which is marked by a locked green gate with the word trail on it. Head out on a doubletrack that skirts the northern margin of Lily Lake. Evidence of beaver activity is present right up to where the road is overlaid with sharp rock and wannabe boulders. Within the first 0.5 mile, a US Forest Service sign reminds you to carry a permit into the wilderness, where no fires are allowed. While you're double-checking

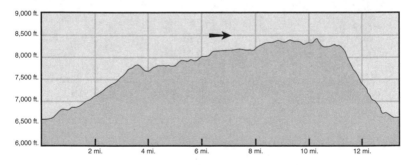

that you have the permit, ensure that you also have a current map of the Desolation Wilderness. It's a busy area with many trails, and consequently you'll encounter numerous junctions. In particular, two critical junctions on this trip are poorly marked. This description will guide you, but a map is always an essential piece of gear.

In just minutes, the road begins climbing across granite boulders and outcrops within sight of a short waterfall behind a summer cabin. Walk about 150 yards north, following the signs posted high in the trees, which ask hikers to stick to the road. A more impressive and enjoyable waterfall splashes 100 feet south of a large runoff stream that crosses the road, about 150 yards after the road turns west. The pools below the falls are suitable for play.

A barn on your left signals your approach to historic Glen Alpine Springs, just 1.1 miles from the trailhead. An information kiosk and the original soda spring mark the trailside site. The trail marker for Grass and Susie Lakes, 200 feet up the forested trail, sends you straight ahead, up the stone steps into the sunlight on a singletrack. The Desolation Wilderness boundary sign at 1.75 miles from the trailhead will remind you about the permit requirement about 100 feet before you encounter an easily accessible spot to refill water bottles.

The rock-and-scree trail leads you across a stream, followed by a restful log in a copse of trees where Grass Lake Trail heads left and Mount Tallac–Susie Lake Trail continues straight ahead. Continue straight northwest, and climb the switchbacks up the face of a granite slope and into the canyon under Gilmore Lake. Head northwest, cross one runoff stream, and then cross Glen Alpine Creek 3.2 miles from the trailhead. Late in the season, the water disappears underground at the trail crossing and reemerges 100 feet downstream but is surely wet here early in the season.

Cross to find a trail marker in a shady copse of lodgepole pines, where you follow the sign to Aloha and Susie Lakes. The path to Dicks Pass leads hikers to Gilmore Lake and Mount Tallac as well. Follow the blazes in the form of a small letter *i* on the lodgepole pines along the rocky trail, past a small seasonal lily pond and a trio of seasonal puddles.

Head downhill to a small flower- and grass-filled meadow. Here, the junction with the Pacific Crest Trail (PCT) leads to Gilmore and Half Moon Lakes on the right and your trail to Lake Aloha on the left. Head left, crossing the stream on the boulder provided there and crashing through the fireweed and corn lily, past the Indian paintbrush, columbine, aster, and clarkia. A U-turn between a fir and pine halfway along the meadow marks the beginning of a brief stairway ascent, past a pair of runoff puddles, up to the ridge 30 feet above Susie Lake's rocky shore. Your route continues on this heading on the opposite shore.

With Jacks Peak looming overhead, traverse the eastern margin of the lake, where many backpackers off-load for the weekend (a good reason to come midweek). Cross the lake's outlet stream; a jumble of timber has created a poor dam but caused an attractive cascade here. Mountain heather and pussytoes cling to the shoreline as you swing around the south end and turn north to circumnavigate the lake. A few more acceptable campsites can be found on the western shore across from the small islands. Depart the lake, ascending on timber and granite stairs, and traverse a small slope graced with heather, lupine, and aster. Cross a meltwater stream before descending to the west on timber stairs as you approach Heather Lake's mouth, marked by a live lodgepole and a standing snag.

Traverse west on this talus-and-boulder slope, remaining well above the northern shoreline. Make sure that no one pulls that "one" rock from the jumble next to your right shoulder. A fair siesta site is located at the west end of the lake amid towering Western hemlocks and lodgepole pines, surrounded by fragrant larkspur, columbine, yarrow, and Indian paintbrush.

Depart Heather Lake, and hike about 250 feet uphill to Lake Aloha. Climb to a meltwater pond, cross a stream, and walk through a willow-clad meadow. Pass under the gray, decaying faces of impressively stout granite outcrops, standing like lithic glaciers. The debris of its terminal moraine shines brightly in the sun at the snout. Rock and timber stairs complete your ascent to the Mosquito Pass Trail junction, which overlooks the northeast corner of Lake Aloha.

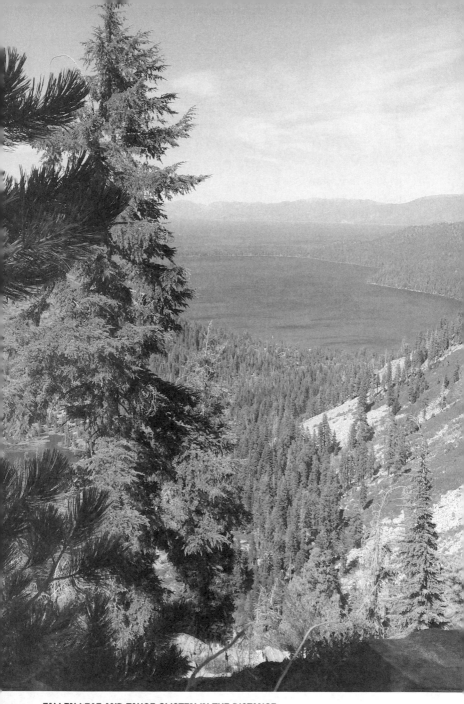

FALLEN LEAF AND TAHOE GLISTEN IN THE DISTANCE.

Ablaze in light most of the time, Pyramid, Agassiz, and Price Peaks shine brilliantly between the Carolina-blue sky and the dazzling waters of Aloha. This is sunglasses territory. Now the route-finding gets easier. With the lake as your handrail on the right, follow the obvious trail across the granite. It sounds implausible that you might go off-route, but just try to walk without constantly staring at the lake and the Crystal Range behind it.

Campsites abound along the lake, and many hikers camp right on the shore and remain somewhat hidden, but it's much better to stay at least 200 feet from the shore. Bivy sites are plentiful and secluded on the north shore, well below and out of sight of the trail. Excellent sites with incredible vistas can be had around and above Lake LeConte, which is 200 feet or so cross-country to the northeast, over a lip and down into a tiny basin overlooking Heather. If you're day hiking, continue southeast toward Lake of the Woods.

The first sketchy junction is nearly 1.5 miles from the Mosquito Pass junction, where the PCT first hit Lake Aloha. Just as you pass the first small copse of lodgepole pines, look for a four-by-four post with no markings in the clearing on the left side of the trail. Heading straight will lead to Lake of the Woods, which does have trails that return to this route, but to follow the described hike, follow the left-hand trail uphill at a slight angle through the lodgepole pines, mistakenly called Tamarack pines by early settlers.

The next 0.5 mile was voted, by a unanimous decision of one, as the most pleasant uphill stretch in the Tahoe area. The trail to Lakes Margery and Lucille and one leading down to Aloha are located within 0.25 mile of each other, followed by another leading to Margery and Lucille again in the same distance. Get ready for more intersections ahead. With many destinations and many people wanting to see them, the Desolation Wilderness is very popular with hikers of all abilities. While day-hike permits are free and valid anywhere, overnight permits require a fee and are restricted by quota throughout the wilderness. In another

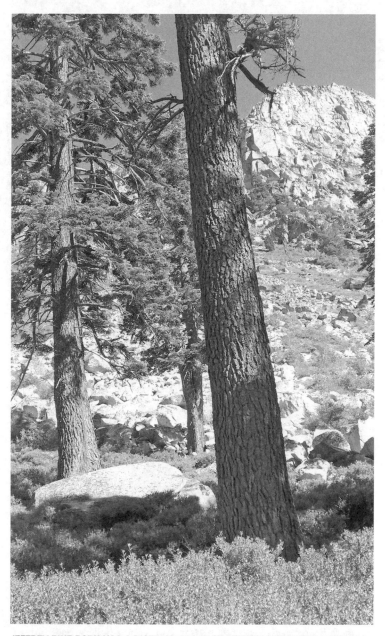

JEFFREY PINE BARK HAS A DISTINCT SCENT OF BUTTERSCOTCH AND VANILLA.

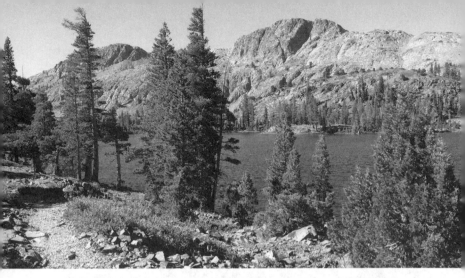

THERE ARE TWO TYPES OF HEATHER AT SUSIE LAKE BUT NONE AT HEATHER.

500 feet, arrive at the top of Haypress Meadows and walk past the junction leading to Lake of the Woods.

Walk about 500 feet farther down-trail to an important trail marker, a crux point at the bottom of Haypress Meadows. Just when you get above Tamarack Lake, look for the junction on the uphill side of the trail that directs you upward to the left to Triangle Lake. Downhill leads to the Echo lakes. Leave the PCT here and traverse directly east across this tree-speckled slope occupied by golden-mantled ground squirrels. Just before topping the ridge, a couple of ancient junipers provide some welcome shade. Take advantage of this vista onto Tamarack, Cagwin, and Ralston Lakes as well as Upper and Lower Echo Lakes.

Descend from the ridge, heading northeast through lodgepole and fir. Go straight past the trail leading to Triangle Lake at the next junction. Echo Lakes are to the right. In 100 yards, be watchful for an unsigned junction. The fork to the right leads to Echo Peak, while your route keeps to the left. The next undulating 0.5 mile of sagebrush, grasses, lupine, and willow takes you to the head of the E-ticket ride, where a sign wisely warns equestrians to turn back, before descending 1,700 feet in 2 miles. Excellent advice. You can ponder that here while taking pictures of Fallen Leaf and Tahoe before beginning a steep descent of Tamarack Creek through a grassy hillside sporting sagebrush and lupine.

The slippery duff trail steepens, and the ravine squeezes in at a point perfect for filling water bottles. Columbine and paintbrush decorate this cool creek crossing. As you hike beneath Angora Peak and Indian Rock, cross the next stream through the brush very carefully. Unseen to the left, on the downhill side, is a steep drop-off with rushing water cascading over it. Pay close attention after that, as you cross a rockfall. The trail curves back to the west and then to the east, where it follows a few scant ducks across a bare outcrop beneath this immense wall of rock. At a point about 15 minutes downhill from the cascade crossing, the trail may seem to vanish, appearing as if you have to down-climb some rock. No climbing is required on this trail. Just walk a few feet straight across the polished rock directly in front of you to spot your route.

When you reach the canyon floor, the track winds past boulders as big as garages, and the vegetation thickens around Lily Lake's inlet streams. Ferns and broadleaf understory make this a pleasantly cool section of trail. But don't be too hasty. It's steep and rocky and wet. The flattening trail and appearance of Cathedral Peak in front of you signal that the road, where you will turn left, is coming up. A quarter-mile lands you in the parking lot again.

Directions

Fallen Leaf Lake Road is located on CA 89, 3.1 miles north of South Lake Tahoe and 24.1 miles south of Tahoe City. Turn from the highway onto Fallen Leaf Lake Road and, in 0.1 mile, take the left fork. Drive 4.7 miles along the narrow and winding road circumnavigating Fallen Leaf Lake, past Tahoe Mountain Road, to the marina at the junction of Fallen Leaf Lake Road and Glen Alpine Road. Bear left on Glen Alpine Road, and follow it 0.6 mile to the trailhead parking lot. The lot is equipped with pit toilets, trash receptacles, and plenty of parking.

Mount Tallac

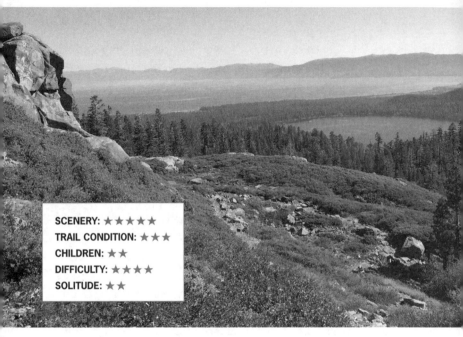

SCENERY: ★★★★★
TRAIL CONDITION: ★★★
CHILDREN: ★★
DIFFICULTY: ★★★★
SOLITUDE: ★★

THE BROAD SLOPE OF MOUNT TALLAC MAKES FOR EASY CLIMBING AND GREAT VIEWING OF FALLEN LEAF AND TAHOE LAKES.

GPS TRAILHEAD COORDINATES: N38° 55.290′ W120° 04.092′

DISTANCE & CONFIGURATION: 9.6-mile out-and-back

HIKING TIME: 7 hours

OUTSTANDING FEATURES: Mount Tallac is a popular trail for one main reason: It has a magnificent vista of Lake Tahoe, Cascade Lake, Emerald Bay, and Fallen Leaf Lake, as well as a view into the Desolation Wilderness with Pyramid Peak, Freel Peak, and Mount Rose on the horizon.

ELEVATION: 6,175′ at trailhead

ACCESS: Depends on snow; permits required for day hiking and overnight camping

MAPS: *Lake Tahoe Basin* (Trails Illustrated 803)

FACILITIES: None

CONTACT: US Forest Service, Taylor Creek Visitor Center, 530-543-2674, tinyurl.com/taylorcreekvisitorcenter

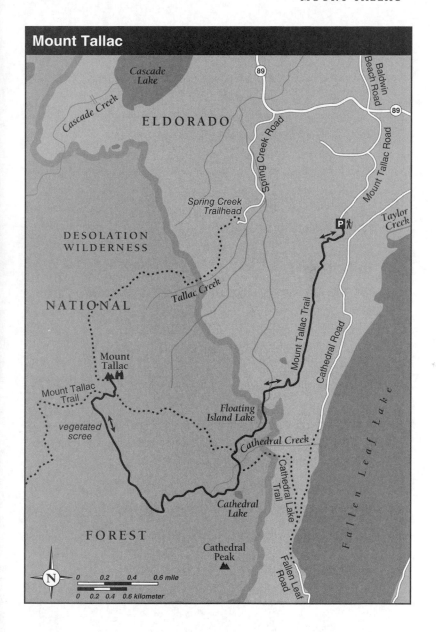

Mount Tallac

Overview

Your path from the Desolation Wilderness Trailhead is a straight-forward march south along a well-defined ridge that offers excellent vistas over the cobalt-blue waters of Fallen Leaf Lake. The views continue as your trail sidles by tree-lined Floating Island Lake, where your final destination's reflection stands out sharply in the placid waters. But right after Cathedral Lake, the bliss ends. The views will distract you from the torturous switchbacks, stairs, and straight-ups leading to a vegetated talus slope capped by Mount Tallac. The memorable photos from the summit are your reward for persisting across windblown slopes and scree-covered trails.

Route Details

Once you've filled out your day-hike permit for the Desolation Wilderness, start down a forest road behind the information kiosk. A conveniently placed signpost assures you that you are on the route to Mount Tallac and gives two reminders: A wilderness permit is needed, and fires are prohibited.

Your trail strikes out to the west, rising quickly in the first 5 minutes through the manzanita and sagebrush. Enter the tree cover to traverse just beneath the crest of a ridge. When your heading turns firmly south, your hike parallels the shore of Fallen Leaf Lake, even though it remains out of sight for the moment. In another 0.25 mile,

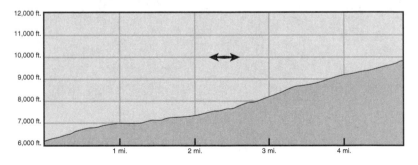

you'll have an excellent vista of Fallen Leaf Lake. Nine years later, some of the damage from the 2007 Angora fire is still visible from here.

As the Jeffrey pines exposed at the top of this ridge begin to warm up in the sun, they release a wonderful butterscotch scent that fills the air for the next 0.3 mile. Here, the vistas of Fallen Leaf Lake persist, and you may lose some time to camera work unless you wait till your return to get glare-free shots. Tree cover thickens as you leave the open vistas behind and head south along the ridge. At a tight stand of six Jeffreys, the gravel-and-dirt trail turns into rocky steps that descend from the ridge. The trail makes several direction changes as you ascend on short switchbacks over gravel then traverse through the pine, fir, and manzanita on your way to Floating Island Lake.

Within an hour of the trailhead and 100 feet before encountering Floating Island Lake, you'll cross the Desolation Wilderness boundary. Standing next to a downed Jeffrey pine, the boundary marker reminds hikers about the need for a permit. Watch for the Spring Creek Trail as it joins yours on the right from the northwest.

Mountain maple, mountain ash, and red fir cover the landscape as you approach Floating Island Lake (where no island currently floats). The view into this lake is mesmerizing, but the tread is rock- and root-encrusted, so watch your step. This oval pond is the perfect spot to reflect on your day's destination. While you're at it, take pictures of Tallac's jagged peak framed in the mirrorlike surface.

Pass by Floating Island's east shore on the rocky trail. As you ascend the stone stairs, the flora's red and gold fall wardrobe is visible among the Western hemlock. Head southwest across the talus slope on this scree-and-gravel trail. Your well-defined trail continues easily across the slope and is crossed by a seasonal runoff stream just before skirting a small knob. A larger stream crossing on the south side of the knob is Cathedral Creek, where logs and rocks assist your crossing.

Ascend southward under the cover of lodgepole pine, and watch for a junction, about 150 paces ahead, with the connector to Fallen Leaf Lake Trail. About twice that many steps after the junction bring you to touch the corner of little Cathedral Lake. This diminutive tarn, lined with talus and scree and decorated with lodgepole pine, Western hemlock, and red fir, is the point where the trail turns west and heads uphill into a broad cirque under Tallac. From here, your climb to the top of the headwall is about 975 feet and should take you about 45 minutes.

The rock stairs, plus the trail repairs and realignment, are a welcome improvement. Still torturous but now shiny, the trail leads up to a vista point—conveniently located next to a solitary juniper flattened in its krummholz attire—just where you need to catch your breath. The view of Cathedral, Floating Island, Fallen Leaf, and Tahoe is one you may want to recall often. When you leave this bliss, a couple of switchbacks will warm you up before going in and out of tree cover.

Switchbacks get thrown out the window as your trail starts straight up the cirque. As you near the headwall, the trail makes a dramatic traverse to the northwest for about the length of a football field before the uphill torment resumes to the south. Just before reaching the plateau, a group of small hemlocks marks an inconveniently large boulder in mid-trail. Remember it for the walk down. But for more memories, watch for Pyramid Peak and Mount Price to appear over your horizon as you approach the lip of this cirque. Vistas from the Tallac Trail marker, just 500 feet distant, are incredible.

Once atop the cirque, you face a broad, open scree field that stretches to the west. This vast plateau slants dramatically away to the west, not steeply, just an enormous mass diving down as Tallac's summit ascends. The soil, though scant and covered with talus, scree, and gravel, is able to produce ground-hugging vegetation such as pussypaws and buckwheat, plus tobacco brush and fireweed. It also supports woodpeckers and golden-mantled ground squirrels.

Make a sharp U-turn to the northwest to begin ascending this massive, tilted block. Traverse the vegetated scree to a small willow- and sedge-covered meadow. The vista in front of you steepens and the trail remains distinct as your only interruption is to detour around a large red fir that has obliterated the trail just 800 feet shy of the peak.

Continue your climb up these gentle slopes where, 300 feet below the summit, your path intersects the route to Gilmore Lake. A wooden post marks this junction, and arrows indicate that you need to go right for the final 15 uphill minutes. As you head east through the stunted lodgepole, watch for the golden-mantled ground squirrels carrying massive amounts of seeds in their cheeks, digging furiously, disgorging their chow, and running aimlessly away.

The trail approaches the base of the rockfall by edging up next to the east face before turning gradually northwest. A few braided trails lead from this point, so look up and pick your route, then see if a trail matches it. The summit of jagged, broken rock affords little room for dallying, as every hiker wants the same view of the lake in his or her picture.

Directions

From Truckee, drive 37 miles south on CA 89 to Mount Tallac Road across from Baldwin Beach Road. Turn right and drive 0.4 mile to the first left turn onto an unnamed road; then drive 0.7 mile to the parking area at the trailhead. From South Lake Tahoe, drive 3.9 miles north on CA 89 to Mount Tallac Road. Turn left onto Mount Tallac Road, and follow the above directions to the trailhead. There are no facilities at this trailhead. As you select your parking spot, be aware that late in the season, the Jeffrey-pine cones that fall from 75 feet up weigh more than a pound.

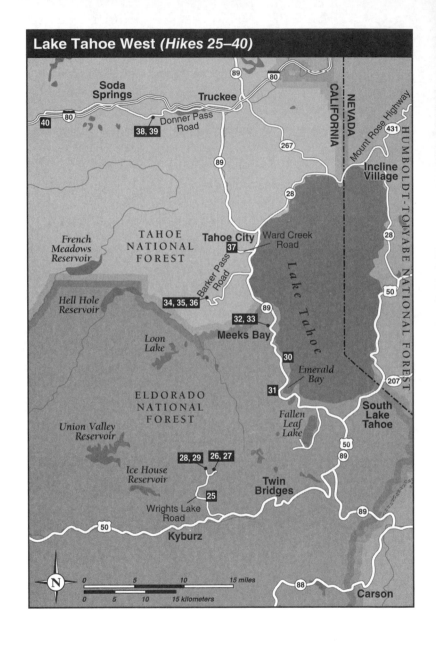

Lake Tahoe West (Hikes 25–40)

Lake Tahoe West

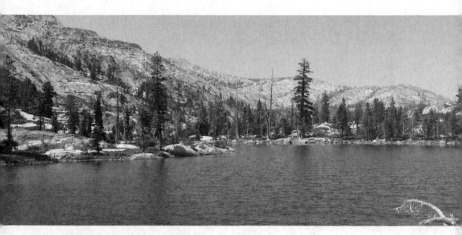

BETWEEN LAKES 2 AND 3 AT 4-Q LAKES *(see Hike 29, McConnell Lake Loop, page 206)*

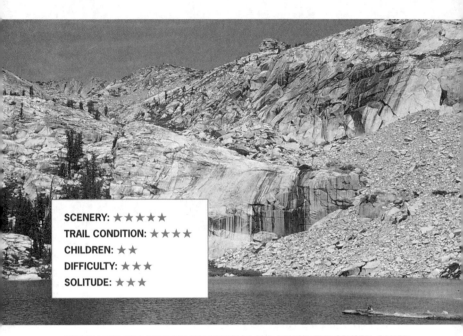

SCENERY: ★★★★★
TRAIL CONDITION: ★★★★
CHILDREN: ★★
DIFFICULTY: ★★★
SOLITUDE: ★★★

LYONS LAKE SITS BENEATH MOUNT PRICE AND BEHIND THE CRYSTAL RANGE.

GPS TRAILHEAD COORDINATES: N38° 48.626′ W120° 14.367′

DISTANCE & CONFIGURATION: 12-mile out-and-back

HIKING TIME: 6 hours

OUTSTANDING FEATURES: Massive granite wall at north end of Lyons Lake; shallow pools along the steps of Lyons Creek; base camp beneath Pyramid Peak

ELEVATION: 6,730′ at trailhead

ACCESS: Depends on snow; permits required for day hiking and overnight camping. Pick up your free day permit at the kiosk adjacent to the trailhead, which is marked by a green gate. Overnight camping permits are available for a fee at the Taylor Creek Visitor Center, 150 yards to the west of Fallen Leaf Lake Road on CA 89, or online at tinyurl.comdwovernightcamping.

MAP: *Desolation Wilderness* (Wilderness Press)

FACILITIES: Pit toilet

COMMENTS: Bring sunglasses and sunscreen.

CONTACT: US Forest Service, Taylor Creek Visitor Center, 530-543-2674, tinyurl.com/taylorcreekvisitorcenter

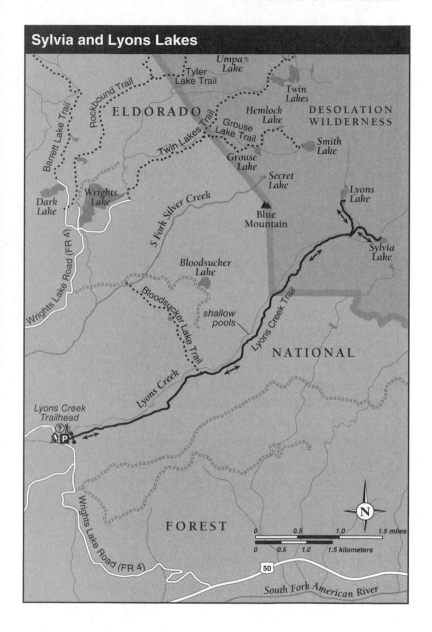

Sylvia and Lyons Lakes

Umpa Lake

Tyler Lake Trail

Rockbound Trail

ELDORADO

Twin Lakes

Hemlock Lake

DESOLATION WILDERNESS

Grouse Lake Trail

Twin Lakes Trail

Smith Lake

Grouse Lake

Barrett Lake Trail

Secret Lake

Lyons Lake

Wrights Lake

Dark Lake

S Fork Silver Creek

Blue Mountain

Sylvia Lake

Bloodsucker Lake

Bloodsucker Lake Trail

shallow pools

Wrights Lake Road (FR 4)

Lyons Creek Trail

NATIONAL

Lyons Creek

Lyons Creek Trailhead

Wrights Lake Road (FR 4)

FOREST

N

| 0 | 0.5 | 1.0 | 1.5 miles |

| 0 | 0.5 | 1.0 | 1.5 kilometers |

50

South Fork American River

Overview

At the end of Lyons Creek Trail, the Desolation Wilderness yields up two of its most beautiful tarns. Sylvia Lake sits beneath hidden Pyramid Peak and makes a great staging spot for a climb to the summit. The rewarding climb to Lyons Lake brings you face-to-face with magnificent beauty—from the flowers at your feet to the towering trees growing out of the sheer granite walls. This moderate hike offers wildflowers, lakes, and gentle streamside pools for hikers' pleasure.

Route Details

Your trail begins to the left of the information kiosk, where you'll pick up a Desolation Wilderness day-hike permit. After filling out the paperwork and checking distances on the map, head generally northeast along the former four-wheel-drive road, passing by an unused but locked gate.

This parklike trail is guarded by barrel-loads of butterflies and a similar number of mosquitoes. It ends and the singletrack begins after about 0.4 mile, just where a pine on the right has tried to eat a metal sign. After about 20 minutes of hiking, you cross the first of many small streams that feed into Lyons Creek to your left.

By mid-June, the corn lilies are popping through the soil, and by the first of July, they are joined by columbine, larkspur, lupine, yarrow, elephant's head, Indian paintbrush, and aster. This colorful

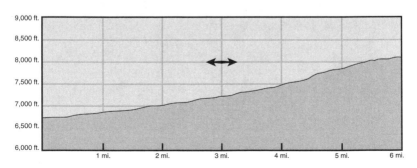

display is a needed diversion because the trail has morphed from pleasant dirt to rocks, boulders, roots, and sand.

Lyons Creek is your "handrail" as you navigate a northeasterly course marked by numerous "blazes" on the trailside trees. Formed in the shape of a small letter *i*, these markers are most often found on lodgepole pines and can take on grotesque attributes as the tree ages.

Your trail will alternate between sand and rock as you pass by the intersection to Bloodsucker Lake Trail, almost 2 miles along. Within minutes, you will be on the margin of a small meadow where delicate five spot and mountain bluebells rub shoulders with sub-alpine paintbrush and corn lily.

Your trail rises ever so gently as you follow it over the next stream crossing, assisted by several large granite blocks. Ignore the mosquitoes here and watch the wandering daisies being mauled by tiger swallowtail and checkerspot butterflies.

As you enter the signed Desolation Wilderness at about 3.5 miles, your rock trail becomes more exposed. You'll cross another stream, moving to the north side of Lyons Creek, within another few hundred feet. The trail becomes significantly rockier as you head uphill. Pussypaws, lupine, and dark-blue camas adorn the trailside, while bluebells and columbine gather near the stream crossings.

Over the next mile, the trail hugs the stream, and you should be able to find several comfortable spots to dangle your toes in the water or sit in a shallow pool as the creek runs across the bare, polished granite.

While the granite wall to the north steepens as the stream chips away at its base, the rocky trail crosses a wide stream just before reaching the Sylvia–Lyons junction. After about 2.5 hours of moderate hiking, spend a few minutes first heading northeast and then swinging around to the southeast to reach placid Sylvia Lake, which is bordered by bare granite on its eastern flank. The lake's west side, shaded by lofty pines and firs, has several highly impacted "sacrifice" campsites that make a great base camp for climbing Pyramid Peak. Use these sites rather than creating more impacted areas.

Return the half-mile to the junction and begin the 400-foot ascent to another glacial tarn, Lyons Lake. The trail heads northeast across lightly wooded terrain to intersect the creek about 750 feet ahead. The rock and sand trail is unrelenting in its effort to shred your calves and thighs, but its 20% grade abates after about 0.4 mile, yielding a beautiful view of a supremely impressive cirque and tarn.

Lyons initially confronts you with a small, picturesque holding pond beneath its 3-foot rock dam. The easiest trail continues past it on the west side of the outlet stream and crosses the dam to the eastern shore, where you can find some suitable campsites on the flat outcrops above the lake.

The shore of Lyons Lake is fringed with a white and pink display of white heather and mountain heather, both of which are abundant in July. Not to be outdone are the Sierra penstemon, the pinemat manzanita, and especially not the anemone sequestered among the rocks and boulders on the east side.

While this hike ends here, adventurous hikers can continue around the north end of the lake and up through the notch leading back to the east and Mount Price followed by Mount Agassiz and Pyramid Peak.

As you switchback down the 400 feet to the trail junction, look in the stream for small trout and on the hillside for star tulip, mountain pride penstemon, and Lemmon's draba.

Directions

From US 50, 5 miles west of Kyburz or 4.1 miles east of Strawberry, turn north on Wrights Lake Road/Forest Road 4 and drive 4 miles to the Lyons Creek Trailhead, just before the ford of Lyons Creek. You'll find parking for about 15 cars on the right. More parking is available across the road or along the road. The trailhead is behind the sign at the trailhead parking lot.

26

Grouse, Hemlock, and Smith Lakes

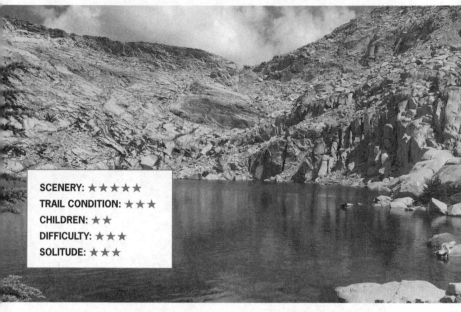

SCENERY: ★ ★ ★ ★ ★
TRAIL CONDITION: ★ ★ ★
CHILDREN: ★ ★
DIFFICULTY: ★ ★ ★
SOLITUDE: ★ ★ ★

SMITH HAS ITS SHARE OF MOUNTAIN HEMLOCK AND SECLUDED CAMPSITES.

GPS TRAILHEAD COORDINATES: N38° 51.029′ W120° 13.573′

DISTANCE & CONFIGURATION: 6-mile out-and-back

HIKING TIME: 3.5–4.5 hours

OUTSTANDING FEATURES: Glacier-polished rock and pristine subalpine lakes

ELEVATION: 6,721′ at trailhead

ACCESS: Depends on snow; permits required for day hiking and overnight camping. Pick up your free day permit at the trailhead kiosk; overnight camping permits are available for a fee at the Taylor Creek Visitor Center, 150 yards to the west of Fallen Leaf Lake Road on CA 89, or online at tinyurl.com/dwovernightcamping.

MAPS: *Desolation Wilderness* (Wilderness Press)

FACILITIES: Pit toilets

COMMENTS: Use sun protection on this hike.

CONTACT: US Forest Service, Taylor Creek Visitor Center, 530-543-2674, tinyurl.com/taylorcreekvisitorcenter

Grouse, Hemlock, and Smith Lakes

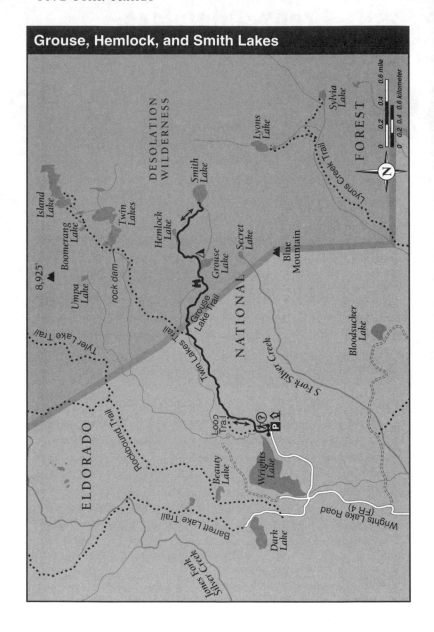

Overview

The short hike to these three beautiful lakes rewards hikers of all ages with stunning vistas down onto Wrights Lake and the Crystal Basin from up on the edge of the Crystal Range. Your hike begins in a flower-filled meadow and includes cascading streams, glacier-polished granite, and snowcapped peaks. This trek is mostly easy but does have some short, strenuous sections to remind you of the elevation.

Route Details

Facing the attractive arched bridge crossing the South Fork Silver Creek, turn slightly right and walk to the information kiosk at your trailhead. Starting from the trailhead at the kiosk, you bypass the Loop Trail and cross the seasonally wet area to the northeast using the foot-bridges. Watch for the sign for Twin and Grouse Lakes to the right.

This wet meadow is filled with wildflowers in the spring. Unfortunately, the ground is also swollen with snowmelt, and hikers are often busier watching their step. Beneath the cover of Douglas-fir and lodgepole pine, you'll pass over a few seasonal streams with the aid of some small footbridges made of either stone or wood. After 100 feet, you'll pass through by a DO NOT ENTER stile for horses. After 0.4 mile, the Loop Trail leads off to the left, and this hike heads to the right, following signs to Grouse Lake.

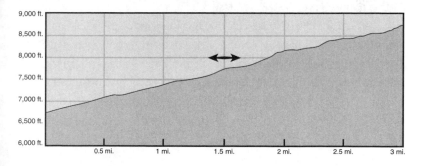

After about 15 minutes of hiking, you'll begin to gain some elevation. The trail is slightly sketchy at first, but rock and boulder steps lead you away from the granite terrain for just a short while and into the trees. Some monster stairs made of boulders will help you ascend a set of switchbacks.

As you reach the 1-mile mark, look for "ducks" marking the trail to the north-northeast on this granite slope. Ducks are, most often, three rocks stacked in a prominent place to help indicate a trail. Here, they line the trail like a sidewalk. In any case, avoid following ducks one at a time; pause, look around, and line up two or three ducks ahead so that you get a sense of the trail, a mental map that will allow you to more enjoyably absorb your surroundings. *Caution:* Ducks can sometimes be misleading, and not all ducks are properly positioned. Hiker beware.

Continuing north-northeast, you'll veer to the right when you reach the end of the granite incline. While the trail is somewhat faint here, you can follow the blazes on the trees, which you may notice as you climb up some exposed roots. In years past, these trail markers (most often a lowercase letter *i*) were scored into the tree bark above eye level. While trail crews no longer create these blazes, they can still be useful for land navigation and route-finding. When you first approach the stream at this point, don't cross it. Rather, continue up the trail to the sign marking the border of the Desolation Wilderness. At this point you've hiked 1.1 miles.

After 1.3 miles, Grouse Lake Trail splits with Twin Lakes Trail. Note that you still have not crossed the stream. As you follow the ducks through this boulder field, notice the weathering of the granite, which exposes these hard, dark inclusions. Ranging from 2 to 12 inches, the inclusions were probably the original rock embedded in the magma chamber where this granite pluton cooled. On the more colorful side, you might spot large clusters of sierra lilies and subalpine paintbrush in this wet area.

Continue straight uphill, somewhat angling across the polished granite, and exit at the top right corner through the pinemat

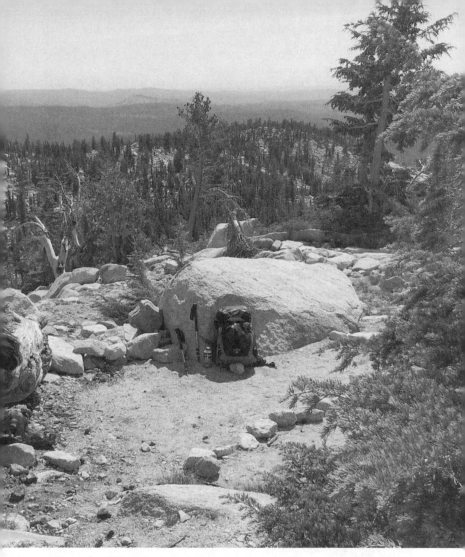

WHEN WINDS TURN THE AIR FRIGID, A SHELTERED SPOT IS PREMIUM TERRITORY.

manzanita. Keep your eye out for ducks as your trail continues trending northeast.

Before the next set of rocky switchbacks, you'll encounter a nice vista of Wrights Lake and the Crystal Basin. You'll recognize the outlet stream for Grouse Lake as it braids out over the trail and cascades downhill to your left. Boulder-hop over this soggy stretch, then climb up through the break on the north side of the lake. If needed, this is a great spot to get out of the wind.

Grouse Lake is rather small, but that allows it to warm up a bit earlier than other lakes. Unfortunately, its rocky shore does not invite much camping. There are a couple of designated camping spots at the northeast edge of the lake, most easily seen as you ascend from the lake on the trail toward tiny Hemlock Lake. If you're inclined to camp, head east-southeast across a low ridge, where you can camp near Secret Lake just beneath you.

Leave the northeast end of Grouse Lake and wind uphill, traversing at an angle toward Hemlock Lake. Notice the very old trail blazes on some very small trees. Despite their small size, these trees have racked up a number of years but have been dwarfed or stunted by the harsh climate (a phenomenon known as the krummholz effect). Without taking a boring from the tree, you would not be able to accurately guess its age.

Winding through some large boulders leads to a wet meadow, where another blaze in front of you points the way to more switchbacks, followed by a fairly level area. Hemlock Lake has a dramatic wall on its northeast shore. The enormous boulders surrounding the lake exhibit the same weathering pattern as that granite wall. Called exfoliation, the pattern is created when rock is peeled off through a process of repeated freezing and thawing of water, which acts as a lever to pry off layers like an onion. While you daydream about that, the camp robbers—Clark's nutcrackers—know how to recognize a tired and hungry hiker. Beware of them while you're snacking here at Hemlock Lake.

As you head toward Smith Lake, only 0.5 mile away, you'll pass some decent campsites on the right side of the trail skirting Hemlock. It's a mere 350 vertical feet to the outlet of Smith Lake, but half of that is in the last 0.1 mile. The views east and north (with the unseen Mount Price in the background) are spectacular. While good camping spots around Smith Lake take some searching, there are several areas where boulders will shelter you from the wind so you can fix a hot drink and a snack before heading back down.

Pay particular attention to the ducks while you walk faster on the way down, as some of them can be misleading. In fact, at some spots along the trail they can be pretty amusing: Some ducks are rather complex, with five or six rocks, while others are just plain casual, with only two. As you enjoy the luxury of walking downhill, take time to notice the polish on the granite at your feet. Stop and look around at the hillsides. The reason you don't see that many trees is that the topsoil was scraped away during the last glacial period and the soil here is fairly new.

Directions

From US 50, the road to Wrights Lake is halfway between Kyburz and Twin Bridges. Wrights Lake Road/Forest Road 4 intersects US 50 4.5 miles from Kyburz and 5.5 miles from Twin Bridges. From the Y in South Lake Tahoe, drive about 4.5 miles to Meyers on US 50 south. Follow US 50 16.5 miles to Wrights Lake Road on the north side of the highway. Turn north and drive 4.1 miles, where you cross Lyons Creek and continue another 4 miles to the lake. You will pass logging pullouts and roads leading left to Icehouse and Crystal Basin.

When you reach Wrights Lake, pass through a gate and a stop sign, where you'll spot an information kiosk on the left. Turn right, heading northeast, on Forest Road 12N23. Drive slowly along this one-lane road beneath tall lodgepole pines 1 mile, passing a group camping area on your right and summer cabins next to the lakeshore on your left. The parking lot is at the end of this road, surrounded by boulders.

Your trailhead is past the gate marked OFFICIAL VEHICLES, which is across from two pit toilets. Walk down that road, and head northwest to a gravel path that leads over to the trailhead kiosk.

27

Island and Twin Lakes

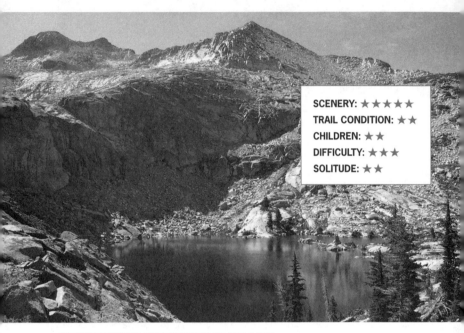

BRILLIANT CIRQUE SURROUNDING ISLAND LAKE

GPS TRAILHEAD COORDINATES: N38° 51.029′ W120° 13.578′

DISTANCE & CONFIGURATION: 8-mile out-and-back

HIKING TIME: 5–6 hours (overnight)

OUTSTANDING FEATURES: Wildflowers scattered across glacially polished granite with peaks above, views below, and several pristine lakes

ELEVATION: 6,721′ at trailhead

ACCESS: Depends on snow; permits required for day hiking and overnight camping. Pick up your free day permit at the trailhead kiosk; overnight camping permits are available for a fee at the Taylor Creek Visitor Center, 150 yards to the west of Fallen Leaf Lake Road on CA 89, or online at tinyurl.com/dwovernightcamping.

MAPS: *Desolation Wilderness* (Wilderness Press)

FACILITIES: Pit toilet

COMMENTS: Use sun protection on this hike.

CONTACT: US Forest Service, Taylor Creek Visitor Center, 530-543-2674, tinyurl.com/taylorcreekvisitorcenter

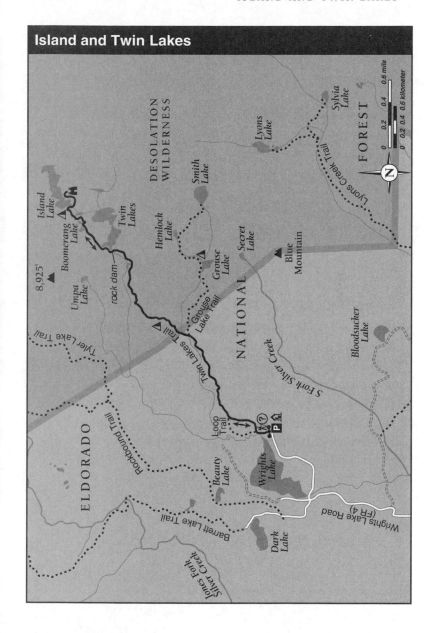

Island and Twin Lakes

Overview

This hike is challenging because of its difficult, flower-lined trail, but its destination is well worth the effort. By continuing past Twin Lakes and ascending to a meltwater lake above it, hikers can escape the crowds and gain fantastic vistas of the Crystal Range, where sunset colors paint the sheer granite walls. Your ascent begins on granite at the edge of a buggy meadow, climbs through a lodgepole pine and white fir forest, follows ducks and blazes across open granite slopes, and crosses streams before ascending a final 200 feet to a pristine bivy site sheltered by a small copse of trees. While descending the 150 feet to Island Lake to regain the trail home past Boomerang Lake and Twin Lakes, you will learn everything there is to know about the lifestyle of marmots.

Route Details

This 3.5-mile trail requires some route-finding skills, so prepare yourself with a map, a compass, and comfortable trail shoes. Using the map, familiarize yourself beforehand with the route and the destination.

Leave the Twin Lakes Trailhead parking lot, pass the gate across the service road, and head to the signed trail that leads to the right to your trailhead. Ignore the picturesque arched footbridge in front of you, and turn right to the informational kiosk. Your trail—Twin

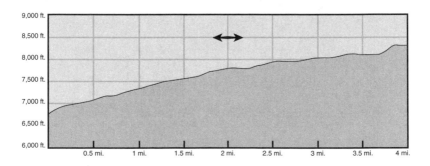

Lakes Trail—begins as you head to the right of the kiosk on the dirt footpath. Small stone or wooden footbridges will help you across the wet spots in this meadow, which is festooned with corn lilies. After a wooden footbridge, watch for the junction of the Twin Lakes Trail with the Loop Trail. The Twin Lakes Trail leads right, where you will begin skirting a granite outcrop.

Mountain pride penstemon adorns each crack and crevice in these large granite steps. Delicate pink pussypaws surround a granite boulder the size of an 18-wheeler. Splashes of yellow are provided by the groundsel, and a handful of star tulips hide among the rocks. At this point, your trail turns from rocky and sandy to forest duff and dirt. Notice the blaze in the shape of the lowercase letter *i* on the lodgepole pine to the left. While this type of blaze is no longer used by the US Forest Service, be alert for it, as the blazes can indicate your correct trail, especially after crossing a stream or granite slope.

Here, under the cover of lodgepole pines and white firs, the trail turns from rocky to rooty. Watch your step as you climb through the boulders, rocks, roots, and a granite outcrop on your right. Early in the season, you may find streams where the trail is supposed to be. Continue climbing the large granite steps until your trail angles off through the lodgepole pines. Keep alert for even ancient blazes on the trees. You'll encounter hundreds of ducks marking the trail, which may be helpful at times, but they also mark alternate trails that you may not want to follow.

Your trail steepens as you hear the meltwater crashing through the chasm north of the trail. Within a few hundred feet, you will encounter the Desolation Wilderness boundary sign. Pass it and continue on the south side of the creek until, in about 300 paces, you arrive at the junction of the Twin Lakes and Grouse Lake Trails, where you are about 1.3 miles from the trailhead.

Your trail continues beneath pine and fir, zigzagging up until you hit a large granite field. Skirt the bottom of this field as you head left, generally northeast. You will cross a small creek just before

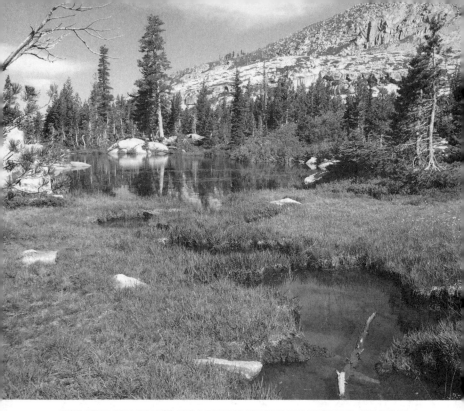

THIS POND AND STREAM ARE A SOURCE OF FOOD FOR MARMOTS AND VOLES.

heading across a short granite slope. Your boulder-lined pathway leads to a small creek crossing.

Continue trending generally northeast across vast granite slopes that will reflect the sun, cooking your body from every direction. Plenty of sunscreen and a brimmed hat are called for on this hike. Keep an eye out for ducks, rocks, and boulders that have been lined up across the glacially polished granite. They serve as convenient "handrails" to keep you within the lines. Gaze ahead for some continuity in these markers because the snow sometimes moves them misleadingly out of place. Other convenient hiker signs are affixed on several lodgepole pines along the way.

The stone underfoot was shaped largely by glaciers and later meltwater. The crescent-shaped divots are called chatter marks—the result of boulders in the glacier's base sticking as the glacier flowed over the bedrock. You will also notice other divots in the stone, this time created by small charges of dynamite. These "petro scars" often mark the correct route when there is no other indicator of the trail.

When your trail levels out at the top of the hill, turn around for a beautiful view of Wrights Lake and the surrounding hills. You'll make a couple of direction changes here as the sandy trail winds along and runs into a chaparral-covered hillside where an indistinct trail made of boulders barges uphill. Initially, your boulder-bordered trail is quite distinct.

Where the wind whips unhindered across this glacially scoured landscape, the lodgepole pines begin exhibiting the krummholz effect. This "crooked stick" effect is the result of dramatic environmental influences on trees, resulting in their stunted appearance. Ground-cover, slope aspect, temperature variation, moisture levels, and wind all have an impact on trees at this elevation.

Your course will head east following the outlet stream from Twin Lakes, South Fork Silver Creek. Pay close attention to your rock-bordered trail, because it will lead you safely and mostly dryly across the stream. The trail passes through several wet areas before the creek crossing. Approaching the lake, your trail will pass over two narrow stone dams to reach the north side; there, your trail continues on the way to Boomerang Lake. In early summer, this is usually a very wet area.

Before you traverse the south edge of Boomerang Lake, notice the white blossoms of pinemat manzanita and the delicate pink blossoms of mountain heather draped between the rocks. To the northwest of this little lake is Peak 8925, triangular and pointed in contrast to its rounded companion just to the east. Watch for the trail ahead as you exit Boomerang Lake. It takes a jog around the smaller ponds before it continues on track to the northeast.

After that you can continue straight ahead to Island Lake. For a secluded night under the stars surrounded by this enormous cirque, there are some suitable campsites. One is on the flat granite overlooking the outlet stream just before the water takes a dive over the slope. Another is on the east side right next to the lakelet underneath a copse of mountain hemlocks. A sheltered bivy site sits on the northwest side as well.

From the point where you encounter Island Lake, you can walk to the southern edge of Island Lake and cross on a stone dam. Explore the north side of the lake, where marmots run in herds of 10–15 at a time. Wonderful vista points abound around Island Lake. Enjoy the hike out with less huffing and puffing.

Directions

From US 50, the road to Wrights Lake is halfway between Kyburz and Twin Bridges. Wrights Lake Road/Forest Road 4 intersects US 50 4.5 miles from Kyburz and 5.5 miles from Twin Bridges. From the Y in South Lake Tahoe, drive about 4.5 miles to Meyers on US 50 south. Follow US 50 for 16.5 miles to Wrights Lake Road on the north side of the highway. Turn north and drive 4.1 miles, where you cross Lyons Creek and continue another 4 miles to the lake. You'll pass logging pullouts and roads leading left to Icehouse and Crystal Basin.

When you reach Wrights Lake, pass through a gate and a stop sign, where you'll spot an information kiosk on the left side. Turn right, heading northeast, on Forest Road 12N23. Drive slowly along this one-lane road beneath tall lodgepole pines for 1 mile, passing a group camping area on your right and summer cabins next to the lakeshore on your left. The parking lot is at the end of this road, surrounded by boulders.

Your trailhead is past the gate marked FOR OFFICIAL VEHICLES, which is across from two pit toilets. Walk down that road, and head northwest to a gravel path that leads over to the trailhead kiosk.

If the trailhead lot is full, you can use the equestrian parking lot as overflow. Both parking lots have a pit toilet. The equestrian parking lot has water.

Lake Lois and Lake Schmidell

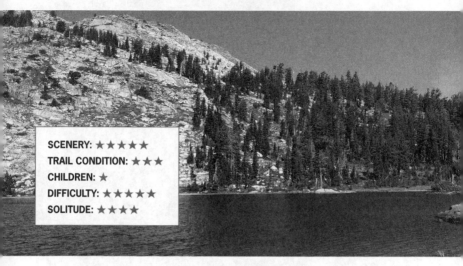

SCENERY: ★ ★ ★ ★ ★
TRAIL CONDITION: ★ ★ ★
CHILDREN: ★
DIFFICULTY: ★ ★ ★ ★ ★
SOLITUDE: ★ ★ ★ ★

LAKE DORIS OFFERS COOL, SHALLOW WATER FOR AN AFTERNOON REFRESHER.

GPS TRAILHEAD COORDINATES: N38° 50.892′ W120° 14.336′

DISTANCE & CONFIGURATION: 18.2-mile out-and-back

HIKING TIME: 10 hours (overnight)

OUTSTANDING FEATURES: Meltwater streams coursing across glacially polished granite that shines even on cloudy days; wildflower displays along every meadow and stream; crossing the Crystal Range to a granite-bound mountain lake

ELEVATION: 6,954′ at trailhead

ACCESS: Depends on snow; permits required for day hiking and overnight camping. Pick up your free day permit at the trailhead kiosk; overnight camping permits are available for a fee at the US Forest Service Pacific Ranger District office in Fresh Pond, east of Placerville on US 50, or online at tinyurl.com/dwovernightcamping.

MAPS: *Desolation Wilderness* (Wilderness Press)

FACILITIES: Pit toilet

COMMENTS: Entry and overnight stays in Desolation Wilderness are quota-controlled by zone. Because Lake Lois and Lake Schmidell are in different zones but only 1 mile apart, I've included route information for both lakes, just in case the zone's quota for one or the other is filled.

CONTACT: Eldorado National Forest, Pacific Ranger District, 530-644-2349, www.fs.usda.gov/eldorado

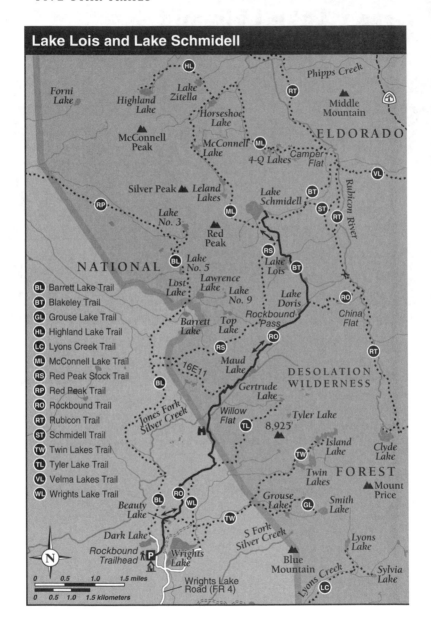

Lake Lois and Lake Schmidell

Forni Lake
Highland Lake
Lake Zitella
HL
Phipps Creek
RT
Middle Mountain
Horseshoe Lake
McConnell Peak
McConnell Lake
ML
4-Q Lakes
Camper Flat
ELDORADO
VL
Silver Peak
Leland Lakes
Lake Schmidell
Rubicon River
BT
ST
RT
RP
Lake No. 3
ML
Red Peak
Lake Lois
RS
BT
NATIONAL
BL
Lake No. 5
Lawrence Lake
Lake Doris
RO
China Flat
Lost Lake
Lake No. 9
Rockbound Pass
BL Barrett Lake Trail
BT Blakeley Trail
GL Grouse Lake Trail
HL Highland Lake Trail
LC Lyons Creek Trail
ML McConnell Lake Trail
RS Red Peak Stock Trail
RP Red Peak Trail
RO Rockbound Trail
RT Rubicon Trail
ST Schmidell Trail
TW Twin Lakes Trail
TL Tyler Lake Trail
VL Velma Lakes Trail
WL Wrights Lake Trail
Barrett Lake
Top Lake
RS
RO
RT
Maud Lake
16E11
DESOLATION WILDERNESS
BL
Gertrude Lake
Jones Fork Silver Creek
Willow Flat
TL
8,925'
Tyler Lake
Island Lake
Clyde Lake
TW
Twin Lakes
FOREST
Mount Price
BL RO WL
Grouse Lake
GL
Smith Lake
Beauty Lake
TW
Dark Lake
Rockbound Trailhead
P
Wrights Lake
S Fork Silver Creek
Lyons Lake
Blue Mountain
Sylvia Lake
Wrights Lake Road (FR 4)
Lyons Creek
LC
N
0 0.5 1.0 1.5 miles
0 0.5 1.0 1.5 kilometers

Overview

"Lake Lois and Lake Schmidell" sounds so friendly and gentle, with a poetic ring to it, but this hike is the opposite of easy. The name of the trail—Rockbound—should be your first clue. Bound on the left, on the right, and to the front by granite (more likely, granodiorite), every step is on rock and more rock. Or so it seems. From either trailhead, gain the Rockbound Trail, which raises you from 6,800 feet to 8,600 feet in 6 miles. The shine of the polished granite is interrupted by sluggish erratics, determined conifers, and stealthy wildflowers. Climb to Rockbound Pass and look out over Rockbound Valley from the crest of the Crystal Range. A short descent on the Blakely Trail brings you to beautiful Lake Lois for a peaceful night beneath an open sky.

Route Details

Take plenty of deep breaths while you're at the trailhead, because there are several times en route when you will audibly gasp at the beauty of the Desolation Wilderness and the Crystal Range. This is a magnificent area and the trail to Lois is exceptional. There are longer hikes than this one—and some steeper—but the trail approaching and climbing to Rockbound Pass has a special degree of difficulty that needs to be taken at a slow, plodding pace.

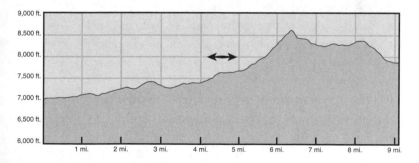

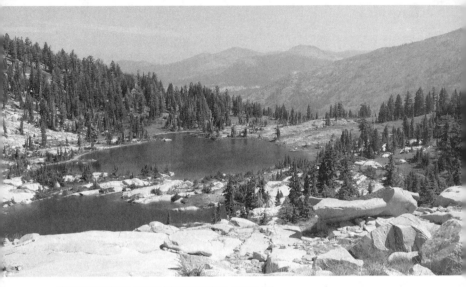

THE VIEW FROM DORIS IS WORTH THE CLIMB UP.

Embark from the trailhead to the right of the pit toilets at the Dark Lake parking lot, under cover of mixed conifers. The duff trail soon turns to a premonition of this route—stairs of boulders and stones—which levels out among shoulder-high boulders within the first 0.25 mile. If you get an early start, the warming sun will toast your back as you take a heading on a predominantly northeasterly line. Ignore the connector trail coming from Wrights Lake as you pass Beauty Lake under lodgepole pine and white fir. The standing snags in the dark, shallow water give the pond a strange beauty indeed. The downed timber in this area has called for the trail tread to be rerouted here.

The trail wraps around Beauty at the signed intersection for an off-highway vehicle (OHV) trail (which leads off to Barrett Lake), where a NO CAMPING sign leans haphazardly against a stout pine on the right. The trail marker sends you along on duff with ferns brushing against your legs and then uphill on a sandy trail to a junction with the Twin Lakes tie trail after an easy 0.9 mile. Walking straight leads to Wrights Lake on the Twin Lakes Trail. The Rockbound Trail continues left on a northeasterly track.

Hustle around the corner, gain a bit of elevation, and within 0.25 mile you will have a grand vista (one of many) of Pyramid Peak, Mount Agassiz, Mount Price, and the massive walls along the Crystal Range. Around you, the towering firs are crowned with upright cones, which, heavy with sap, sparkle like disco balls in the bright sunlight.

You'll encounter another junction just an hour out from the trailhead. This trail, also from Wrights Lake, is the final leg from the Twin Lakes Trailhead parking area. If you decide to start there instead, you would initially walk north-northwest from the Twin Lakes Trailhead 0.4 mile and then continue on a paved road 0.2 mile. At that point you will be on the trail, meeting at this junction after about 0.75 mile of legwork.

After you depart this junction heading northeast, watch for rapid direction changes as you cross the bare rock. Manzanita flourishes in the larger crevices while penstemon creeps into tiny vertical or horizontal cracks in the rock. Before you reach the Desolation Wilderness boundary, an enormous panorama opens before you. Enjoy this vista, looking at the cobalt-blue sky wrapped across the polished granite littered with erratics (boulders dropped in situ by melting glaciers) of all sizes that add texture to this living topo map.

But don't get lulled into missing the trail. You'll be saying "Huh?" while looking around in a circle if you lose track of the pathway on the rock. Instead, use HUH to your advantage—heads-up hiking, that is. Watch for every sign possible by being alert for footprints in the sand, ducks made of three rocks, blazes on trail-side trees (particularly at creek crossings), and "handrails" made of rocks or boulders lining the trail. Be cautious about following erroneous tracks and ducks that you won't know are off-track if you go too far, too fast. Slow travel and heads-up hiking will keep you on track.

The junction to Tyler Lake is about 0.5 mile past the last junction. There, amid a lodgepole grove, you turn left and the Tyler Lake trail heads straight. Per the trail marker, Rockbound Pass is only 3 miles on. (*Only?* Bwa-ha-ha-ha.) The pleasant duff-and-dirt trail beneath the Western white and lodgepole pines here leads to a substantial stream crossing 5 minutes ahead. Roll around the rounded knob of rock to your west before crossing a ravine onto more bare bedrock.

After 3 miles on the trail, your vista is blue sky and hills, granite and conifers. Descend briefly from a small saddle, and anticipate yet another humongous vista just around the corner. The sand on the granite creates very slippery footing along here, but blast marks made by trail builders help you follow the path. Cross a meltwater stream to discover a broad vista that's expansive in breadth and height and glaringly bright with the midmorning sun climbing into a cobalt-blue sky. Make sure you bring along plenty of pixels for this hike. Here, it's easy to imagine the routes of the glaciers, as perhaps three of them flowed over top of everything you see in front of you toward this spot.

Descend to the Jones Fork of Silver Creek, and cross on either the boulders or on the log. It may not always be windy here, but don't be surprised if you see the bark being blown off the trees. It's time to get set for the next stream, though, as its waters cascade past. Cross on the boulders that have been set up to help you cross safely. Look around for the foot-tall red-orange pinedrops that grow beside the trail here. They are a parasite (like snow plants and sugar sticks) that feeds not on plants but rather on the fungi that feed on other plants. Nature indeed abhors a vacuum.

In another 5 minutes, about 2.5 hours after embarking, you get a spectacular look at Pyramid Peak. The trail is smartly lined with rocks heading up the side of this glacial escape route. You can see textbook evidence of glacial activity in the polished surfaces of the granite and in the chatter marks, which are the curved smiles on the bedrock where a rock in the ice was stuck on the bedrock and chipped at it. The curve is usually convex in the direction from which the glacier flowed.

Before reaching Willow Flat, you must cross a small hill. Take this moment to be awestruck by the vastness and immensity of the glacially sculpted terrain before you. You can see chatter marks on

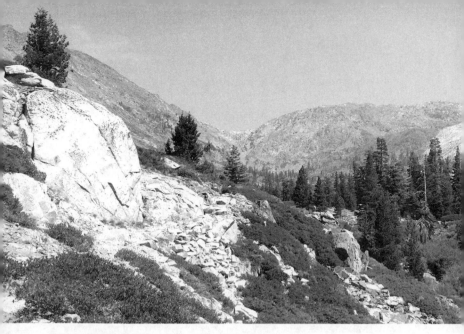

THE ROCKBOUND TRAIL LIVES UP TO ITS NAME.

the granite to the left as you walk down the stairs toward Willow Flat, where you'll find aspen trees, corn lily, ferns, paintbrush, and leopard lily. The trail rises 1,325 feet from Silver Creek to the pass over the next 2.75 miles. You're on the easiest part at this point, because 925 feet of that occurs in the last 1.25 miles.

Another couple of runoff streams cross your path, and Lorquin's admiral butterflies pass going the opposite direction, probably heading to Willow Flat for lunch in their preferred breeding grounds among willows. Your second crossing is next to a large, angular piece of quartz-encrusted granite. Watch the ferns; they hide their roots, which easily grab hikers' ankles.

Back on granite, you start doing a serpentine walk, passing up the turnoff that heads southwest to the Red Peak Stock Trail. Climb a set of stone stairs. The ducks and rocks bordering the trail mark the path well so that you can see the sights. The strange-looking dark spots in the granite are just inclusions of granitelike rock that existed in the magma chamber before the molten pluton rose and the rock simply fell into the molten magma.

Follow boulders, rocks, and drill holes to keep up with the trail as it winds northeast. The juniper offers refreshing shade, and the views into Maud Lake's outlet canyon are easy on the eyes as well. Traverse along Maud, which is at about 7,725 feet.

Cross two causeways past Maud's inlet streams and climb across the meadow above the lake; then head for the white pine and the granite stairs. Only 925 feet remain to climb over the next 1.25 miles, and the views are spectacular the entire way. A welcome and venerable-looking juniper shades you at the most appropriate point on your climb to Rockbound Pass. When you reach the pass, you can set your altimeter according to the sign nailed to a red fir atop the pass at 8,650 feet in elevation.

A little display of heather accompanies you down the trail toward Lake Doris, while a verbal greeting from several marmots shouldn't surprise you as you descend past chatter marks on the rock beside you. Don't start counting the stairsteps, as they will just make you want to stay out and not go home instead of climbing them. (I didn't even try to count.) The gray rock is colored by penstemon and paintbrush, and hemlock shades your tread. Step across a few meltwater streams as you approach Doris and its inlet culvert. This moist area is thick with mauve-hued mountain heather. Cross more meltwater streams as you climb away from the lake on a gravel trail with tiny lupine on its margins. From this vantage, it appears as if there could be a fair bivy spot at the southwest corner, close to the pass, or in the trees at the northwest corner.

Within moments, you will pass the trail to China Flat that leads down into Rockbound Valley. At this point, it's time to join the Blakely Trail leading to Lake Lois and Lake Schmidell. Veering to the left side of the canyon, traverse to the northwest across a broad meadow of willow and sedges flanking a small runoff pond. Lake Lois is visible now in the distance.

Before descending to the lake level, look for an excellent bivy site to the left of the trail among the rocks at the northeast edge of the lake. On the chance that the quota here is filled, try for a permit to Lake Schmidell, where there appear to be plenty of fish.

To get to Schmidell, descend to the meadow at the north end of Lois, and skirt the marshy land by traversing to the east. Cross the dammed outlet, and follow the faint trail across the rocks to its exit from the lake, heading uphill once again. The singletrack is easily visible as it leads to Lake Schmidell. Again bypass a junction with the Red Peak Stock Trail halfway to Schmidell. Pass another floral magnet as you head downhill on a pretty chunky trail. This is not the most pleasant part of the trail but your rest at Schmidell is just ahead.

At the junction of the trail to Leland Lakes, the McConnell Lake Loop, turn right to stay on the trail to Schmidell. Leave this view of the lake, and descend a bit toward the granite outcrops concealing the waters from sight. Bivy sites can be found at the southwest and southeast corners of the lake on granite, and passable tent sites are located across the outlet dam.

Directions

From the Y in South Lake Tahoe, drive about 21.5 miles west on US 50 to Wrights Lake Road on the right, 4.5 miles west of Strawberry. If you're coming from the west, Wrights Lake Road is 35.8 miles from Placerville and 4.9 miles east of Kyburz via US 50. Be prepared for the turn, which comes up suddenly at a curve in the road.

Drive 8 miles to the Wrights Lake Visitor Center, just past the equestrian parking lot, and then turn left to the Rockbound Trailhead at Dark Lake. Drive 0.4 mile to the trailhead parking area, where pit toilets are available.

If that lot is full, you can park at the Twin Lakes Trailhead by turning right at the visitor center onto FR 12N23 (straight if coming from Dark Lake parking) and driving 1 mile past the summer cabins to the end of the road to the trailhead parking lot. Pit toilets are available there. If both lots are full, you can use the equestrian parking lot, which has water and pit toilets.

McConnell Lake Loop

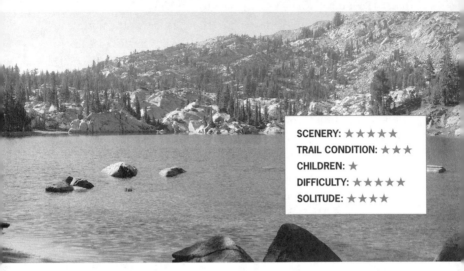

> **SCENERY:** ★ ★ ★ ★ ★
> **TRAIL CONDITION:** ★ ★ ★
> **CHILDREN:** ★
> **DIFFICULTY:** ★ ★ ★ ★ ★
> **SOLITUDE:** ★ ★ ★ ★

LELAND LAKES OFFER A SECLUDED GETAWAY FOR SUN AND SWIMMING.

GPS TRAILHEAD COORDINATES: N38° 50.892´ W120° 14.336´

DISTANCE & CONFIGURATION: 26-mile balloon loop

HIKING TIME: 2 nights

OUTSTANDING FEATURES: Pass by or visit any one of 13 beautiful mountain lakes; fill every photo card with enormous vistas of the Crystal Range; discover new geologic wonders; and wander past meadows filled with willows, wildflowers, and butterflies. Nights are filled with stars and wind.

ELEVATION: 6,954´ at trailhead

ACCESS: Depends on snow; permits required for day hiking and overnight camping. Pick up your free day permit at the trailhead kiosk; overnight camping permits are available for a fee at the US Forest Service Pacific Ranger District office in Fresh Pond, east of Placerville on US 50, or online at tinyurl.com/dwovernightcamping.

MAPS: *Desolation Wilderness* (Wilderness Press)

FACILITIES: Pit toilet

COMMENTS: Entry and overnight stays in Desolation Wilderness are quota-controlled by zone. Because Lake Lois and Lake Schmidell are in different zones but only 1 mile apart, I´ve included route information for both lakes, just in case the zone´s quota for one or the other is filled.

CONTACT: Eldorado National Forest, Pacific Ranger District, 530-644-2349, www.fs.usda.gov/eldorado

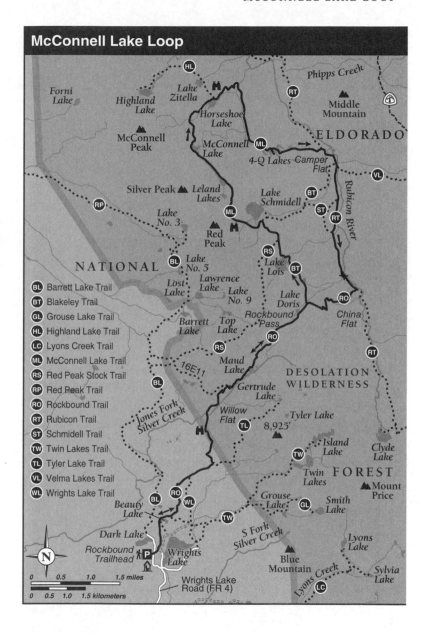

McConnell Lake Loop

Phipps Creek

Forni Lake

Highland Lake

Lake Zitella

Horseshoe Lake

Middle Mountain

ELDORADO

McConnell Peak

McConnell Lake

4-Q Lakes Camper Flat

VL

Silver Peak Leland Lakes

Lake Schmidell

Lake No. 3

Red Peak

RP

Rubicon River

NATIONAL

Lake No. 5

Lawrence Lake

Lost Lake

Lake No. 9

Lake Lois

Lake Doris

China Flat

Rockbound Pass

Barrett Lake

Top Lake

Maud Lake

16E11

Gertrude Lake

DESOLATION WILDERNESS

Willow Flat

Tyler Lake

8,925'

Island Lake

Clyde Lake

Jones Fork Silver Creek

Twin Lakes

FOREST

Mount Price

Beauty Lake

Grouse Lake

Smith Lake

Dark Lake

Rockbound Trailhead

Wrights Lake

S Fork Silver Creek

Lyons Lake

Blue Mountain

Sylvia Lake

Wrights Lake Road (FR 4)

Lyons Creek

Trail legend:
- BL Barrett Lake Trail
- BT Blakeley Trail
- GL Grouse Lake Trail
- HL Highland Lake Trail
- LC Lyons Creek Trail
- ML McConnell Lake Trail
- RS Red Peak Stock Trail
- RP Red Peak Trail
- RO Rockbound Trail
- RT Rubicon Trail
- ST Schmidell Trail
- TW Twin Lakes Trail
- TL Tyler Lake Trail
- VL Velma Lakes Trail
- WL Wrights Lake Trail

N

| 0 | 0.5 | 1.0 | 1.5 miles |
| 0 | 0.5 | 1.0 | 1.5 kilometers |

Overview

If you have the time and can handle the vertical miles, this may just be one of the most exciting, challenging, and beautiful hikes in the Tahoe region. Depart from Wrights Lake on Rockbound Trail, and plan for a night at Lake Lois or Lake Schmidell. Climb west above Schmidell, and begin a clockwise, descending circuit to several inviting lakes on the McConnell Lake Trail, which (I'm certain) was built by, and not improved since, the Spanish conquistadores. Cross the nascent Rubicon River in Camper Flat, and ascend the Rubicon Trail to its junction with Rockbound Trail leading up to Lake Doris. Return for a cold beverage at the trailhead.

Route Details

Since you're here, you must have made it up and over Rockbound Pass, as described in the previous hike.

Make sure that you have a map and compass and know how to use them before heading out on this loop. At times you will have a grand vista, and other times you will be searching for stream crossings under cover of forest or following scant markers over granite outcrops. Aside from that cautionary word, this is one of the best areas for hiking in the Tahoe region.

You have some choices for your first night's campsite. Lake Doris has good sites, but my vote is for staying at Lake Lois, just for the vistas across the Rubicon Canyon to Middle Mountain. If you are

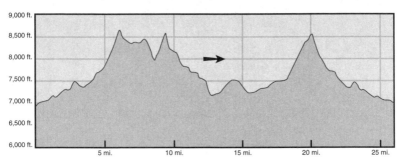

unable to secure a permit in this zone, then the next logical campsite would be a mile away at Lake Schmidell. Climb away from Lake Lois, and descend about 550 feet to its granite-lined southeast shore. Look for the junction of the trail to Leland Lakes as you near the lake level.

The best sites to set a bivy are on granite at the southeast end of Schmidell. These are reached by heading to the left when the trail hits the hemlock-shaded outcrops. After a night spent with the winds howling down the east face of Red Peak, regain the trail for a wilderness hike. Head back to the junction leading off to the southwest, and traverse about 200 yards to a stream crossing. After using the boulders to get across the cascading water, climb smartly out of the ravine and ascend steeply above the south end of the lake. There's an impressive vista to the north if you need an excuse to catch your breath.

Your track turns uphill and heads northwest 0.25 mile before another meltwater stream crosses it, cascading down the steep slope at your left shoulder to resume its downward plunge at your right boot after crossing the narrow trail. Watch and listen uphill for any rocks that might be tumbling down this steep watercourse as it fills Schmidell then continues to the Rubicon below. Climb out of the ravine, past rangers' buttons and lupine. A clearing just past a copse of hemlocks and pines marks the spot where the trail turns brutally uphill for 100 vertical feet.

This trail may not be all that enjoyable for hikers who have difficulty with exposed heights, but it isn't dangerous. You will ascend about 450 feet more to the saddle overlooking Leland Lakes, essentially passing behind the cirque that stands above Schmidell. Marmots may watch and verbally pass judgment as you traverse the willow-dotted slope. The trail is mostly visible, but vigilance is key as you sometimes must follow scant but accurate ducks.

Cross another stream on your way to the saddle. In a moment, the gravel trail leads through willows and pinemat manzanita up to a rockfall. From there, ducks mark the trail as it winds through a meadow to a hemlock-shaded saddle looking down on Leland Lakes. This pair of blue gems is set amid green Western hemlocks, which seemingly outline the shores of the twin tarns cut into granite bedrock.

Not to be outdone in steepness, this trail leads impatiently downhill—nicely lined as it leads away from the saddle, then becoming fairly scrabbly before turning seriously steep—requiring near-technical skills to negotiate some of the steps. With granite walls above, the descent abates about 50 feet above the first lake. Walk through some boulders, and follow the trail as it turns away from the lake. The trail, spongy in early season, sounds a hollow note after summer heat has sucked all moisture from it. It wanders on a northerly course past the first lake and turns northwest to approach the larger tarn. A surprise is in store as you find a small sandy beach with a nice picnic spot adjacent to it among some trees. Vistas along the lake's wide, sandy trail through the granite are plentiful.

The trail's environs become ravinelike as you descend away from the second of the Leland Lakes. A boggle of downed trees will keep you alert for ducks. The trail maintains a northwest heading along the lake's outlet. Pass a shallow meltwater pond on the left and some garage-sized mountain debris on the right. Lots of rocks assist the next stream crossing before you barge through the willows and heather and into a large meadow. The lake's southern margin is fringed by young lodgepole pines, and the trail, now the size of a rabbit track, edges to the granite wall above the west side of the lake.

With Silver Peak on your left, start out on the half-mile downhill to McConnell Lake. Your trail is quite indistinct over the granite and even as it enters the trees, so stay vigilant for ducks and blazes. Although you're looking for a lake, as shown in blue on the map, McConnell seems less like a lake and more like a succession meadow despite, or maybe because of, its small marshy area at the northwest corner. Looking back at the small lodgepole pines moving into the area from the south, it looks as if the meadow first filled with silt and grasses and then willows before allowing the conifers to take over.

The indistinct trail around McConnell will present a challenge to anyone not paying strict attention to the trail and its signs. Winding through trees and over fallen logs, it persists northward toward a wall of boulders. One last walk through the lodgepole pines, and you start ascending across granite, following the accurately placed ducks. Keep high on the wall, and then descend at the north end, following ducks between wet meadow and dry granite.

Crash through the willows that camouflage a drop-off into the next stream and then one more stream before you head across granite to the shade of a short stretch of conifers. Presently, the mystery of the hour is what happens to the stream that bounds down and then disappears beneath your feet. A gradual descent with overwhelming vistas will erase all memories of the next 0.25 mile heading into Horseshoe Lake. Some small ducks lead around and through a gaggle of downed timber. Follow them closely, and continue northeast to slide around the north end of Horseshoe, passing an interesting lodgepole pine whose trunk emerges from the ground twice. It's a great place to take a nap near the western shore, but it's too close for a camp. Besides, fetching water is difficult here.

Climb away from Horseshoe Lake, following ducks across the granite, and soon encounter a junction with the trail to Lake Zitella, a compact tarn sited just 120 feet uphill. You head to Camper Flat on the trail to the right. Notice the lodgepole pine with the blaze— a lowercase letter *i*—carved into its bark. Above the blaze, bolted to the conifer, is a sign declaring HAZARDOUS FOR STOCK TRAVEL. A quick note of thanks for not being a cow or horse, and down you go, some 200 feet to Four-Q Lakes. Walk straight across the sandy path and up a granite outcrop, where you have to stop because of the enormous, eye-filling panorama ahead of you.

Follow the ducks as the trail disappears over the hill, staying high on the granite slope, to traverse along the east-facing slope. An amazing vista awaits as you approach a spot overlooking the Rubicon Valley. Marked by three prominent lodgepole pines separated from a venerable juniper by two boulders, the stout limb of the juniper catches you just before you are, seemingly, about to step over a precipice into the ether.

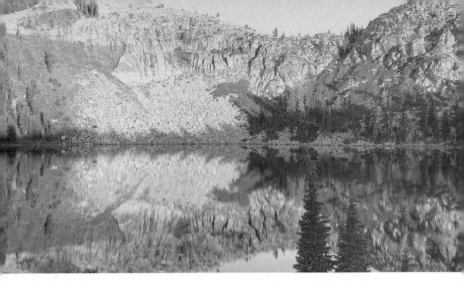

MORNING SUN BOUNCES OFF THE GRANITE SURROUNDING LAKE SCHMIDELL.

Your route-finding skills will come into play as you head downhill to Four-Q Lakes. Look for obvious signs such as ducks, blazes, footprints in sand, dropped bits of trash, and broken sticks or twigs, which can easily keep you on the trail across many types of terrain. You may strain a bit to follow the trail as you make several crossings of the Rubicon's tributaries. On the way to the crossing of Schmidell's outlet stream, descend about 375 feet, following the trail about 0.4 mile to the east. The route is sketchy here and the ducks plentiful through the meltwater ponds and streams throughout this stretch of the young Rubicon. Where you cross is not critical. Walk east just far enough to find a safe crossing, and then make a sharp right turn to the southwest.

The trail, once again outlined with ducks, stretches south on a sandy surface between rock outcrops. Follow the rock piles through the blowdown, even straight uphill. About a mile of traveling to the south, up this tributary of the Rubicon, leads to the first of the Four-Q Lakes. Climb across outcrops, and follow the ducks as you pick your way through a stand of lodgepole. A huge wall of granite stands to the west, and your trail continues uphill through the trees to the southeast. A brief but serious uphill climb steps you up to the corner of the westernmost lake. It's a nice spot beneath the trees—right off the trail and too close to the lake for camping—to filter water and grab a snack.

Regain the trail, which climbs slightly to overlook this and the next lake from about 50 feet above the shore level. Continue trending east, almost contouring above the lakes. Avoid descending prematurely to the next lake; instead, turn slightly uphill to the northeast, where you'll soon overlook the next two lakes and the granite isthmus between them. When you come abreast of it, turn and walk south to several excellent bivy sites on the granite. These are two of the most secluded and picturesque lakes in the Desolation Wilderness, according to me. Sunset and stars have nothing on sunrises here. All of them are wonderful, colorful, and memorable. The hiking time from the previous night's bivy was about five hours.

Return to the trail, refreshed and ready for some descending and climbing, then more climbing and more descending, and then home. Zigzag after the ducks, and contour along to a rocky crossing of another isthmus between two more Four-Q Lakes. The trail changes direction shortly after leaving the last lake's shore. Continue to pay close attention even though the trail becomes more distinct.

Travel a mile from the second lake's bivy site, and you may see a chute carved in granite by rushing water. This is difficult trail to follow but the ducks remain accurate. After a more gentle descent, cross another stream on your way to Camper Flat. A sign facing east cautions riders TRAIL IMPASSABLE TO HORSES 1 MILE BEYOND FOUR-Q LAKES. Equestrians ought to believe that.

Descend a bit more to Camper Flat, where you'll need to watch for a large log on which to cross the stream. Make a sharp left across the creek when your trail is blocked by branches. Cross easily on this large log, and turn right once on the other side. The path is now a sweet trail—soft, wide, and easily navigated—that roughly parallels the curving stream. Just after a side trail to a spring, you will encounter the junction with the trail leading uphill to Lake Schmidell. Ignore this trail and one more leading to Schmidell. Your path heads toward China Flat but ascends to Rockbound Pass before that.

However, in 100 yards or so, the trail to Middle Velma Lake intersects yours. Continue uphill to the right as if you were going to Lake Aloha. Whereas the trail around the loop to the Four-Q Lakes was rather hectic and required full attention, this trail heads south through a conifer forest for the next mile along a placid, well-marked dirt-and-duff trail lit by the sunlight filtering through the tree crowns. As the trail comes adjacent to the Rubicon, finding water to filter is easy. A hundred yards south of gathering water is another junction leading uphill to Schmidell. Continue ahead, immediately cross the trout-bearing creek, and veer slightly southeast under forest cover.

Runoff streams now add some texture to the trail. Continue south through the broken forest until you take a left jog at a small meadow with a lone pine at its south end. With the Rubicon gaining strength to your left, you'll cross a few runoff streams feeding it from your right. First up is a stone bridge, followed by a causeway through a wet meadow of corn lilies, then a quick crossing followed just as fast by another with a dirt-and-stone bridge. After 200 yards you'll encounter another crossing of moderate difficulty followed 100 yards on by one that's much more impressive. Small meadows of corn lily and lupine push the trees back from the trail on your way to the next junction, 500 feet southeast.

Right leads uphill to Rockbound Pass; continuing ahead leads to Lake Aloha. Head right and get ready for your final climb of about 880 feet to the junction of the Rockbound and Blakely Trails. White firs provide welcome shade, even at noon, and the many blazes will keep you on route. Cross an open area of broken red, gray, and black rock in the midst of the trees. Wolf lichen adorns even the standing snags and adds a new shade of green to the forest.

The wind plays havoc with trees as they grow here in the Desolation Wilderness, stunting their height, shortening their limbs, exposing roots, and generally making bonsai trees out of any conifer in its path. Just about 500 feet below Lake Doris is a fine example of this krummholz effect—literally, "bent wood." Two magnificent firs display the force of the wind here: One has been split in half, and the other so windswept and snow-shaped that its lowest limbs actually wrap around the tree before reaching skyward.

A few runoff streams create the moist, meadowlike open areas that support lupine, aster, paintbrush, corn lily, and butterflies. Sometimes a causeway will keep your feet dry crossing these areas. At the last such spot on this uphill, a solitary granite boulder takes a position at the base of the meadow. Fir and hemlock trees sport blazes to guide you across the top of the field and up to the junction where you will head southwest to Rockbound Pass.

The stone stairs at the south end of Doris assist you to the pass. On the way in, it seemed as if there were only a few stairs down. Now the count is several hundred. Make your way up the stairs, no matter how many, and enjoy the vista. Your return path and all of its terrain are laid out ahead of you and all of it (well, almost all) is downhill.

Directions

From the Y in South Lake Tahoe, drive about 21.5 miles west on US 50 to Wrights Lake Road on the north side of the highway, 4.5 miles west of Strawberry. If coming from the west, Wrights Lake Road is 35.8 miles from Placerville and 4.9 miles east of Kyburz via US 50. Be prepared for the turn, as it comes up suddenly at a curve in the road.

Drive 8 miles to the Wrights Lake Visitor Center, just past the equestrian parking lot, then turn left to the Rockbound Trailhead at Dark Lake. Drive 0.4 mile to the trailhead parking area, where pit toilets are available.

If that lot is full, you can park at the Twin Lakes Trailhead by turning right at the visitor center onto FR 12N23 (straight if coming from Dark Lake parking) and driving 1 mile past the summer cabins to the end of the road to the trailhead parking lot. Pit toilets are available there. If both lots are full, you can use the equestrian parking lot, which has water and pit toilets.

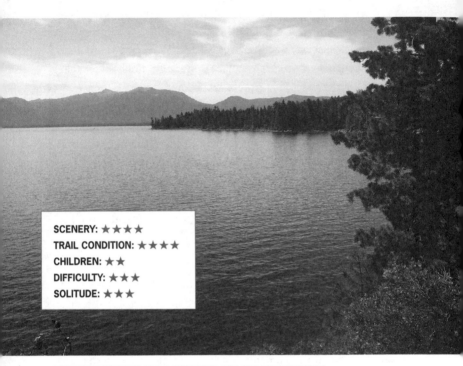

THE RUBICON TRAIL DISPLAYS MILES OF LAKE TAHOE VISTAS.

SCENERY: ★★★★
TRAIL CONDITION: ★★★★
CHILDREN: ★★
DIFFICULTY: ★★★
SOLITUDE: ★★★

GPS TRAILHEAD COORDINATES: N38° 59.913′ W120° 05.860′

DISTANCE & CONFIGURATION: 9.4-mile out-and-back with alternate starting points

HIKING TIME: 4–5 hours

OUTSTANDING FEATURES: A lighthouse, a historic mansion amid majestic trees, sandy beaches, and enormous vistas of the crystal-blue waters of Lake Tahoe and Emerald Bay

ELEVATION: 6,300′ at trailhead

ACCESS: Depends on snow; $6 day-use fee

MAPS: *Lake Tahoe Basin* (Trails Illustrated 803)

FACILITIES: Pit toilets, water at trailhead

COMMENTS: Bring sunglasses and sunscreen.

CONTACT: D. L. Bliss State Park, 530-525-7277, tinyurl.com/dlblissstatepark

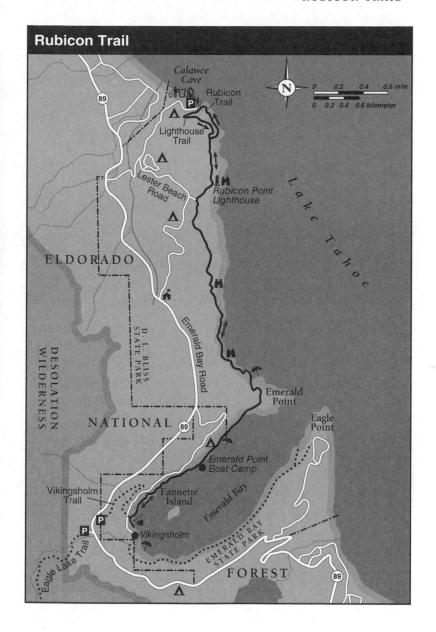

Overview

Hikers on the Rubicon Trail will be treated to spectacular scenery on this fairly moderate trail that begins with a short side trip to a historic lighthouse (plus a great vista) and ends with a visit to a renowned residence nestled among magnificent Jeffrey pines at the head of Emerald Bay. Your trail starts out with a few uphill switchbacks to reach its high point near the historic Rubicon Point Lighthouse, then descends to Emerald Bay, where the highlight is Vikingsholm, a Depression-era mansion. Breathtaking views are common within the first 2 miles, as your trail either looks out on the lake or precipitously down on its shore before entering the cool shade of the Jeffrey pine forest surrounding Emerald Bay. Curious hikers who brought along binoculars will have clear views of Captain Dick's Tomb on Fannette Island.

Route Details

The trailhead begins just past the campgrounds in the day-use parking lot at Calawee Cove. Toilets, water, and trash facilities are available in this parking lot. The trailhead sign is visible at the south end of the lot.

Within the first 100 feet, you will have a choice of two trails. Heading straight south will take you along and above the shoreline on the Rubicon Trail. The described hike starts out on the Lighthouse Trail, which makes a U-turn heading uphill to the historic Rubicon Point Lighthouse. (That sounds a bit grandiose, but I don't want to spoil the surprise: You may be "whelmed," but not overly so.) Ascend

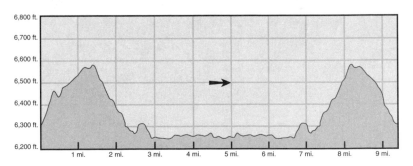

a couple of moderate switchbacks, climbing above the parking lot through a pine-and-fir forest to reach the monument describing the lighthouse and its role in Lake Tahoe's history. The lighthouse itself is about 75 feet downhill and can be reached by a side trail.

From the vista point on the trail past the lighthouse, hikers can get a wonderful panorama from South Lake Tahoe up to Kings Beach, with snowcapped peaks in the background along the entire vista. Genoa, Monument, and East Peaks all stand out against the azure sky. At the junction 500 feet ahead, your trail will continue south while the trail to the north is an alternate trail on which you can return, as shown on this map.

June is a great month for flowers around Tahoe. The shady Rubicon Trail is splotched red by snow plants under the pines and accented by yellow-capped woolly mule's ears along Emerald Bay.

After about 1.25 miles on the trail, you arrive at a junction with a road end where there is some parking for the alternate Rubicon Trailhead. You're about 2.5 miles from Emerald Bay Boat Camp, 3.5 miles from Vikingsholm. Another vista point lies 0.7 mile ahead along this sand-and-duff trail, which is often surrounded by greenleaf manzanita and lined with fragrant lupine.

The Rubicon Trail is regularly maintained, and evidence of that is clear along here, where the manzanita has been cut back and boulders repositioned. The hillsides have been thinned and cleared of underbrush and dead and downed trees in order to reduce the forest's vulnerability to catastrophic wildfires, such as the Angora fire of 2007.

Enjoy the gentle slope as you descend nearer to lake level only to climb back up to cross a stream shooting across the trail. More thinning operations are evident as you approach Emerald Point. You will see a broad, flat area—an impromptu beach—just before zigzagging through the trees across the point. You'll find more tempting beach sites within feet of the trail as you turn southwest toward your destination.

The trail becomes somewhat obscure when it passes through the Emerald Point Boat Camp, but careful attention to signs will keep

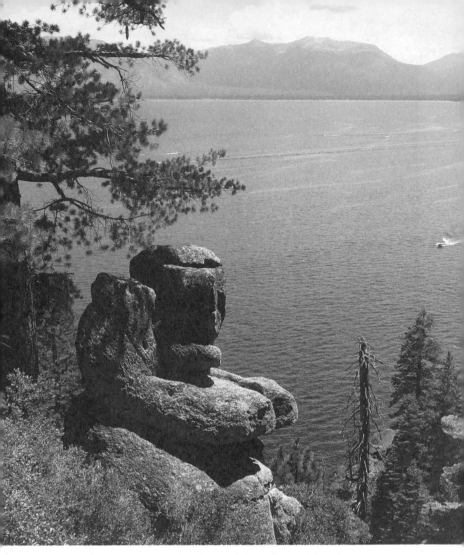

GRANITE MOUNTAINS, MAJESTIC PINES, AND DEEP WATER—TAHOE

you on track. The trail tends to the lakeside just past the boat ramp. Now your level trail is within view of the lake, Fannette Island, and the tour boats that churn around it. On the Vikingsholm Trail, your stream crossings can be made on wooden footbridges.

If you have binoculars, you'll be able to make out the rock structure near the summit of the island. That is the erstwhile tomb of Captain Richard Barter ("The Hermit of Emerald Bay"), which he built for himself while serving as the caretaker for the cottage owned by Ben Holladay ("The Stagecoach King"). He finally needed to use it in October 1873, when he was outrun by a storm on the lake and slipped beneath its surface in 1,400 feet of water off Rubicon Point. The island was formerly referred to as Dead Man's Island.

Nestled among the big trees is Vikingsholm, a grand home built in 1929 and donated to the state park system a quarter of a century later. The building was designed to fit in its surroundings without disturbing the landscape. You can tour the house and grounds, picnic at one of the many tables, or swim in the ice-cold water. Feeding wildlife is discouraged. Restroom facilities are located on the hillside behind the house. You can reach the Vikingsholm parking lot by climbing the stairs and path beyond the mansion up to CA 89.

On your return to the trailhead, follow the trail to the junction of the Lighthouse Trail (uphill) and the Rubicon Trail (straight ahead). Whichever one you took on the way in, try the other on the way out. The Rubicon Trail will carefully guide your steps around the face of boulders that are exposed to the water's edge below. Chain fencing and solid-rock stairs will help you along this section. Four vista points along the trail are worth every pixel.

Directions

Starting at the Y in South Lake Tahoe, drive north on CA 89 about 11.5 miles to the entrance to D. L. Bliss State Park on the right. Drive past the visitor center to the entrance kiosk, where you can self-pay the $6 day-use fee; then continue to the day-use parking lot.

An alternative is to park at the Emerald Bay State Park lot, about 2.75 miles before D. L. Bliss State Park. From this direction, your trail would begin with a 0.7-mile descent to Vikingsholm from CA 89 before hiking the Rubicon Trail in reverse.

Eagle Falls–
Velma Lakes Loop

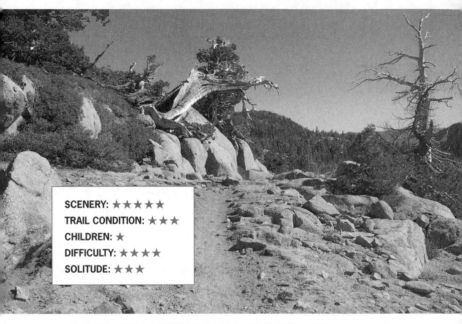

SCENERY: ★★★★★
TRAIL CONDITION: ★★★
CHILDREN: ★
DIFFICULTY: ★★★★
SOLITUDE: ★★★

STONE AND SAND DOMINATE THE TRAIL ABOVE DICKS LAKE.

GPS TRAILHEAD COORDINATES: N38° 57.118′ W120° 06.811′

DISTANCE & CONFIGURATION: 10.8-mile balloon loop

HIKING TIME: 5–6 hours

OUTSTANDING FEATURES: Bridge the creek with snowmelt water crashing over rocks in a wild cascade; pass five beautiful lakes with dramatic backdrops; travel in lush, mixed-conifer forests; and cross erratic-ridden granite bedrock polished smooth by glacial mud.

ELEVATION: 6,609′ at trailhead

ACCESS: Depends on snow; permits required for day hiking and overnight camping. Pick up your free day permit at the trailhead kiosk; overnight camping permits are available for a fee at tinyurl.com/dwovernightcamping.

MAPS: *Lake Tahoe Basin* (Trails Illustrated 803)

FACILITIES: Pit toilet, water, picnic area

CONTACT: US Forest Service, Lake Tahoe Basin Management Unit, 530-543-2600, www.fs.usda.gov/ltbmu

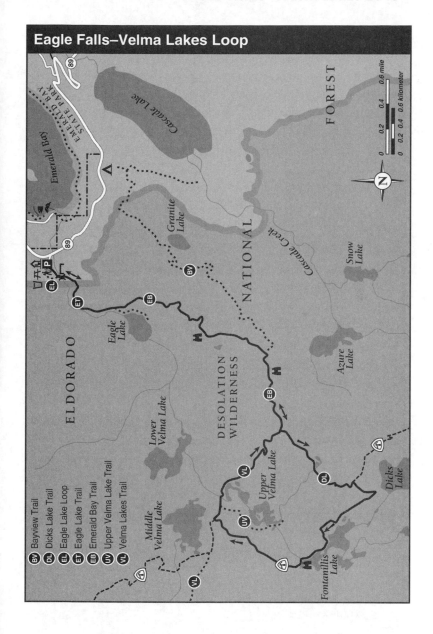

Eagle Falls–Velma Lakes Loop

BV Bayview Trail
DL Dicks Lake Trail
EL Eagle Lake Loop
ET Eagle Lake Trail
EB Emerald Bay Trail
UV Upper Velma Lake Trail
VL Velma Lakes Trail

Overview

This is a popular trail despite being incredibly rocky, but even that makes it an interesting trip. Glacial action was an evident agent of geologic change here, and every rock reveals it. The initial 2.5 miles are strenuous in that your elevation gain is about 1,550 feet—without letup.

Once you see Eagle Lake, you know that more like it must be better. And they are. Velma, Dicks, and Fontanillis Lakes are all amenable getaways for a quiet lunch or an overnight bivy. From Dicks Lake, it's downhill almost all the way back to the trailhead.

Route Details

Walk past the circle in the parking lot, and go up the granite steps to the trailhead kiosk to complete a day-hike permit. Overnight permits are necessary and available at US Forest Service ranger stations. The broad timber-and-sand path leads up and away from the kiosk. A sharp left turn at the outset sends hikers up steps to a junction of the Eagle Lake Loop and Eagle Lake Trail. Follow the trail to the left past buckbrush and huckleberry oak, manzanita and willow, where aspens shake in the canyon breeze. You can rest beneath a venerable spreading Western juniper, on a bench made for eight overlooking the water crashing down the V-shaped ravine.

Continue up the stone stairs to the right, past another vista point and past the Eagle Loop Trail that joins from the right. This

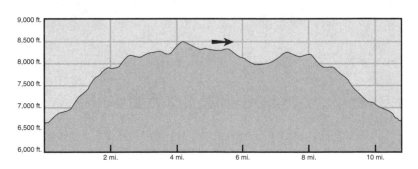

hike takes the trail downhill to the left toward the bridge and Eagle Lake. A stone causeway precedes the bridge where you cross and reach a jumble of rock at the other end. Turn south for 100 yards, and cross into the Desolation Wilderness. Right in the middle of the rock stairs is your reminder about the permits that rangers always seem to want to see. Turn west through the trees to navigate around a small knob for the next 0.25 mile. This uphill traverse crosses a granite slope, then turns south and follows the creek uphill.

As you approach the spur trail to Eagle Lake, the air is filled with the crisp melody of aspen and the fragrant butterscotch scent of Jeffrey pine. Take the right fork at the signed junction, and walk about 150 yards to an overlook of this pretty tarn, graced with a petite island topped by five firs. The north shore offers some areas to sit and snack or contemplate. There are excellent vistas of the lake and its surrounding monoliths from the trail heading uphill. In fact, these changing vistas actually pull hikers uphill, making the slow going quite tolerable.

Sierra penstemon liven the trailside rock clusters with their scarlet outbursts. Chinquapin and huckleberry crowd and claw at your knees from time to time. Cross over a small rockfall among some broken Jeffrey pines just short of 7,400 feet of elevation. From a granite outcrop with a scant view of the lake, descend on a duff-and-dirt path, cross a runoff stream, and then switchback to the south. Climb up some boulder stairs that are easy if your knees are 4 feet off the ground.

Keep aware over the next 200 yards of many short switchbacks, as the scant trail is marked with rocks, ducks or sticks, or not at all. Soon walk across a sandy trail with a copse of lodgepole pines to your left and polished granite to your right. Climb across the granite to the southwest, and then make a loopy ascent to go around a knob. When you reach a small saddle, just before your trail turns south again, your reward will be incredible vistas, including peaks: Phipps to the northwest, Dicks to the south, and Jakes to the north (named for a general, a sailor, and a skier).

Traverse this steep slope about 0.5 mile to the south, losing and gaining a bit on the way. When you reach the decaying granite, be alert for ducks, which will guide your way. Two hundred yards ahead is the junction with Bayview Trail. Turn right, heading west and crossing a spur where another spectacular vista emerges. Dicks Peak and Mount Tallac stand out to the south from this viewpoint. Hike west, descending slightly, across the granite slope among lodgepole, Western white pine, and Western juniper, for another 0.5 mile, where you will encounter an important signed junction.

This new junction marker is about 3.2 miles from the trailhead, at about 8,200 feet in elevation. The trail to Velma Lakes takes a right turn to the northwest; the trail described here departs to the left, southwest. On your way to Dicks Lake, you should practice HUH—heads-up hiking—because the trail becomes somewhat indistinct and cruddy going across rocks and roots. A rock-and-sand causeway helps you cross a seasonal wetland or pond, and a little farther down-hill the trail crosses another few small streams draining the larger pond to the left.

Ahead await 300 feet of switchbacks up granite slopes. What better way to start than with stairs made of local material? As you walk along the switchbacks, observe the scratch marks made by rock embedded in the glacier passing over the granite. The smiley-face cuts are chatter marks, where an embedded rock got stuck and plucked out a piece of granite. These marks indicate the direction that the glacier flowed. This area is easy to navigate if you stay on top of it. If you lose track of the trail, stop and regain your bearings, including your last certain location. Then look for ducks or other trail signs: Footprints, rocks in a line, blazes, dog prints, bits of trash, broken sticks, and flowers are all good indicators if you lose your path momentarily.

If you ever feel totally lost, however, have a seat and think about the humor of the situation for 5 minutes. That should relax you enough to enable you to recall the last known place where you had good trail and then carefully retrace your steps to that point, if possible. If not, then relax and think of your plan that you prepared for this event. No sweat. And that won't happen anyway, because you prepared with other navigation tools and this guidebook.

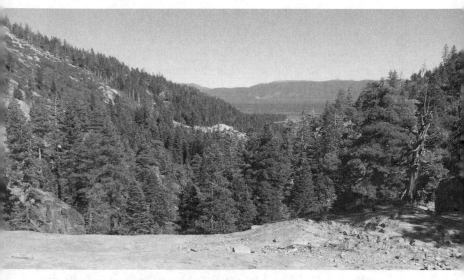

DESCENDING TOWARD EMERALD BAY AND LAKE TAHOE

When you reach the saddle, the trail junction marker stands out just 200 feet to the east. Continue east from there if you want to climb across Dicks Pass or go to Dicks Peak. But if you want to go to Dicks Lake, then you must turn right at the marker. The trail is clearly defined with shattered granite blocks and erratics the size of Hummers as you walk among lodgepole and hemlock. Six minutes down the trail brings you to Captain Richard Barter's namesake swimming hole, where the trail leads down to the outlet from this junction with the trail to Fontanillis Lake. Several secluded bivy sites dot the north shore. Vistas to the southwest over this lake are fantastic.

From the junction marker beneath the hemlock that lost its twin long ago, follow the trail to the right downhill to Fontanillis Lake. The sandy trail heads northwest and is caught between the bedrock hills overlooking Middle Velma on the right and the erratics littering the area around the shore. The trail passes a stagnant pond on the left and, after another wet area, slides up next to the lake. Walk along the lake's heather-laced shore past the outlet before you veer away to the north. It was too wet, too rocky, or too close for any bivy site to be very good.

As you cross the outlet stream amid stands of larkspur, pause to get a view of Lake Tahoe. Follow the trail as it ascends the ridge in front of you, and then descend its west flank to the northeast. The trail is distinct but runs through a debris field of shattered rock and splintered wood. Step across a runoff stream, descending into its ravine, and traverse the opposite bank through red fir and hemlock. The trail remains clear despite the blown-down giants all around.

The cones of the fir glisten with sap as they stand erect at the crown. The firs are also decorated with wolf lichen, catching the sun and adding a fresh green to the forest. Continue downhill through massive blowdowns on a very comfortable duff trail. The junction with the Velma Lakes Trail stands in a copse of hemlocks and firs.

The marker at this junction states that Phipps Pass heads to the left and Bayview Trail is to the right. This route goes right, but there are any number of bivy and tent sites between this junction and 2,000 feet west at the Phipps Pass junction.

Some are within trees, and others are on granite but still secluded. Sunrise on Middle Velma should not be missed. It is a glorious event of color and stillness.

In the middle of the afternoon, a sooty grouse scurries around a hemlock on the duff trail. Woodpeckers hammer, and the wind silently lifts butterflies over the trail. The silence is broken by the male sooty grouse vocalizing during its display. The loud thumping echoes all around the open space just before the Upper Velma junction. Pass by that trail and continue east, crossing the wide outlet stream from it on a convenient log. Climb away from that, and skirt another pond before crossing broken granite to the marshy northern end of that fractured body of water.

Ascend stone stairs to start walking past the shore on a sandy trail across broken granite and shady lodgepole pines. Practice HUH—heads-up hiking—again along here. The trail can morph from distinct to not there in a blink. Watch carefully for all the usual trail signs. Ahead of you is an array of switchbacks and squiggles that haul you about 250 feet uphill across polished and weathered granite. The trail of both stone and timbers is very well constructed. Pass a sandy stretch and it's not yet ready for prime time.

At the next, previously visited, junction, your homeward trail leads to the left rather than returning to Dicks Lake. The next junction, 0.75 mile ahead, returns to the trailhead via Eagle Lake Trail to the left. The Bayview Trail heads right and descends 2.8 miles to the Bayview Trailhead. If another car were available, that would make an excellent loop as well. Without an extra vehicle, this might not be practical. CA 89 is not the easiest road to walk, even for that short distance.

Turn left onto the Eagle Lake Trail, and begin your descent to the trailhead.

Directions

The trailhead parking lot is located at the large curve in CA 89 directly above Vikingsholm, 8.5 miles north of South Lake Tahoe. If coming from Tahoe City, drive 18.6 miles and turn right at the entrance driveway. Parking is available on the road, but more space and facilities are down the driveway. Pit toilets, a picnic area, and water are available. A $5 fee is required for each day parked—if you're doing an overnight, make certain to enclose the right amount. An annual pass for parking around the lake costs $25 and is available from Lake Tahoe Basin Management Unit facilities. It's very useful if you're hiking more than four times from any of the popular trailheads.

32 # Genevieve and Crag Lakes

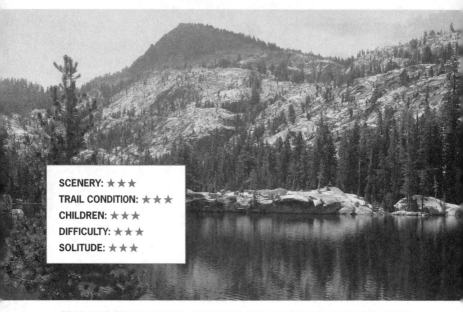

SCENERY: ★ ★ ★
TRAIL CONDITION: ★ ★ ★
CHILDREN: ★ ★ ★
DIFFICULTY: ★ ★ ★
SOLITUDE: ★ ★ ★

CRAG LAKE OFFERS FISHING AND PICNIC SPOTS ALONG ITS SHELTERED SHORE.

GPS TRAILHEAD COORDINATES: N39° 01.608′ W120° 08.704′

DISTANCE & CONFIGURATION: 11.4-mile out-and-back

HIKING TIME: 4–5 hours

OUTSTANDING FEATURES: Butterflies and hummingbirds will blast from flower to flower as they accompany you up this moderate trail to two scenic subalpine lakes.

ELEVATION: 6,215′ at trailhead

ACCESS: Depends on snow; permits required for day hiking and overnight camping. Pick up your free day permit at the trailhead kiosk; overnight camping permits are available for a fee at the Taylor Creek Visitor Center, 150 yards to the west of Fallen Leaf Lake Road on CA 89, or online at tinyurl.com/dwovernightcamping.

MAPS: *Lake Tahoe Basin* (Trails Illustrated 803)

FACILITIES: None

CONTACTS: US Forest Service, Lake Tahoe Basin Management Unit, 530-543-2600, www.fs.usda.gov/ltbmu; Taylor Creek Visitor Center, 530-543-2674, tinyurl.com/taylorcreekvisitorcenter

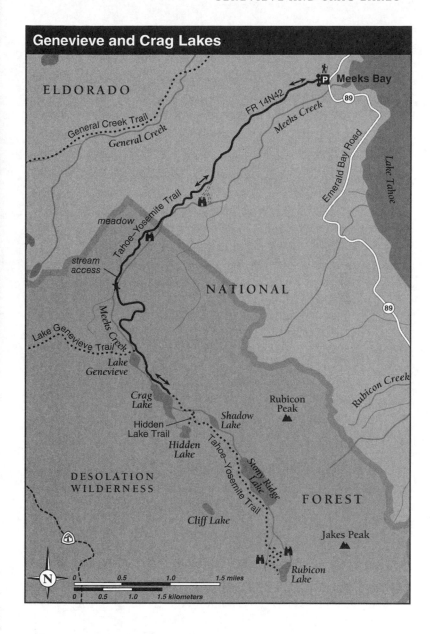

Genevieve and Crag Lakes

ELDORADO

General Creek Trail

General Creek

FR 14N42

Meeks Creek

Meeks Bay

P

89

Emerald Bay Road

Lake Tahoe

Tahoe–Yosemite Trail

meadow

stream
access

NATIONAL

Lake Genevieve Trail

Meeks Creek

Lake
Genevieve

Crag
Lake

Hidden
Lake Trail

Hidden
Lake

Shadow
Lake

Rubicon
Peak

Rubicon Creek

89

Tahoe–Yosemite Trail

Stony Ridge Lake

FOREST

DESOLATION
WILDERNESS

Cliff Lake

Jakes Peak

Rubicon
Lake

N

0   0.5   1.0   1.5 miles

0   0.5   1.0   1.5 kilometers

Overview

This gentle trail leading to a string of scenic subalpine lakes is part of the Tahoe–Yosemite Trail. With only 1,200 feet of elevation gain over moderate terrain, you don't need to exert a lot of energy to enjoy these backcountry vistas in the Desolation Wilderness.

Route Details

From the dirt lot, your path starts on Forest Road 14N42, which begins behind the locked gate marked TRAIL. This dirt doubletrack is your path for the first 1.5 miles. A singletrack begins at the signpost for the Tahoe–Yosemite Trail. A reminder that wood fires are not allowed has been posted as well. After a long, exposed initial stretch of uphill trail, you'll spot a refreshing trailside spring nestled in a shady setting.

Over the next mile, your rocky trail will elevate you about 500 feet. The ridgeline that looms about 1,000 feet over your right shoulder separates the General Creek drainage from the Meeks Creek drainage. That ridge is your handrail, and you'll follow it southwest until you make the turn southeast farther up Meeks Creek heading to the lakes.

On the way, you'll approach Meeks Creek and find a display of pussytoes, Indian paintbrush, lupine, and Sierra fireweed beneath a canopy of pine and fir. After 2.25 miles of hiking, you'll cross the

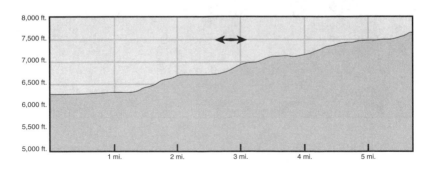

Desolation Wilderness boundary, where your shady, duff-covered trail is often crowded by ferns, columbine, and aster. The sign is a reminder that you need a paid wilderness permit if you intend to camp overnight and a free day-hike permit otherwise. Before you hit your first switchback, you'll pass a dry meadow on a sandy trail where several of the ponderosa pines have had their trunks snapped or crowns blown off by wind or snow.

Climb above the creek, where boulder steps and the exposed roots of ponderosa pine help you up the switchback. Indian paintbrush adds color to the pinemat manzanita that's shared by butterflies and hummingbirds. As you round the large knob to your left, red fir trees border this stream where it is level enough for small pools to form. One mile after entering the wilderness, cross Meeks Creek on a substantial footbridge before making a detour to the east. Just as your route turns southeast approaching Lake Genevieve, you'll have a good vista to Lake Tahoe.

Your sandy trail soon turns rocky, and the last steep uphill before reaching Lake Genevieve has been eased with some steps hammered into the granite. At the top of this little rise, you'll have a pleasant vista in front of you, with diminutive Lake Genevieve on the west side of the trail. Some highly impacted sites at the north end of the lake should be used for picnics and conversation points, as they're too close to the lake to be suitable for camping.

The path keeps you high around the unapproachable south end of Genevieve and continues 0.25 mile to Crag Lake. A sandy trail leads you about halfway along Crag Lake's eastern shore. There, you can snap excellent pictures from its pine-dotted western shore. Continue southeast past the impacted picnic areas and a large rock outcrop where you have the most beautiful vista of the lake reflecting a granite peak.

Cross the stream flowing out of Shadow Lake, and come to the junction of a trail leading to Hidden Lake. You can end your uphill portion of this hike with a secluded swim. Beware of afternoon thunderstorms, which are highly predictable in the summer.

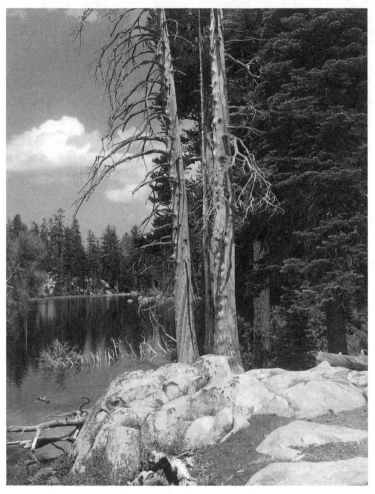

TINY GENEVIEVE LAKE OFFERS A WELCOME PAUSE ON THIS PLEASANT TRAIL.

Directions

The Meeks Creek Trailhead is 11.5 miles south of Tahoe City on CA 89. The trailhead parking lot is on the west side of the road, across from Meeks Bay Campground and Marina. Park in the small dirt lot, which has room for about 10 cars. There are no facilities here. Additional parking can be found along CA 89.

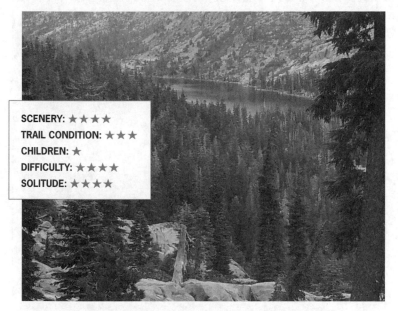

STONY RIDGE LAKE IS IN VIEW AS YOU DESCEND FROM RUBICON LAKE.

GPS TRAILHEAD COORDINATES: N39° 01.608′ W120° 08.704′

DISTANCE & CONFIGURATION: 16.4-mile out-and-back

HIKING TIME: 4–5 hours (overnight)

OUTSTANDING FEATURES: Hikers can find seclusion while visiting five mountain lakes where butterflies enjoy the all-you-can-eat buffet of wildflowers; the trail is shaded by tall pine and fir.

ELEVATION: 6,215′ at trailhead

ACCESS: Depends on snow; permits required for day hiking and overnight camping. Pick up your free day permit at the trailhead kiosk; overnight camping permits are available for a fee at US Forest Service or Lake Tahoe Basin Management Unit visitor centers, or online at tinyurl.com/dwovernightcamping.

MAPS: *Lake Tahoe Basin* (Trails Illustrated 803)

FACILITIES: None

COMMENTS: An approved bear canister is required in most areas of the Desolation Wilderness, including Rubicon Lake.

CONTACT: US Forest Service, Lake Tahoe Basin Management Unit, 530-543-2600, www.fs.usda.gov/ltbmu

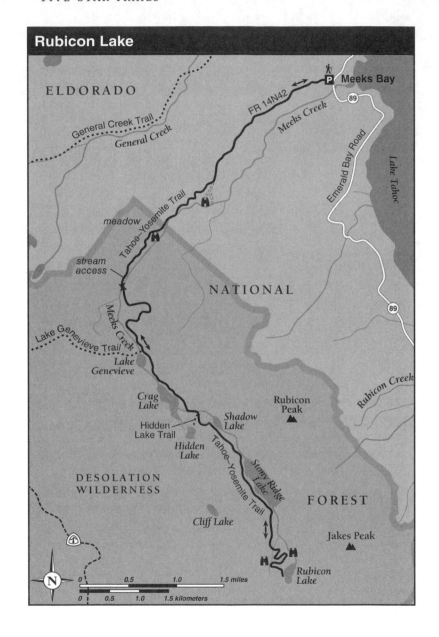

Rubicon Lake

ELDORADO

General Creek Trail

General Creek

FR 14N42

Meeks Creek

Meeks Bay

89

Emerald Bay Road

Lake Tahoe

Tahoe–Yosemite Trail

meadow

stream access

NATIONAL

Lake Genevieve Trail

Meeks Creek

Lake Genevieve

Rubicon Creek

Crag Lake

Shadow Lake

Rubicon Peak

Hidden Lake Trail

Hidden Lake

Tahoe–Yosemite Trail

Stony Ridge Lake

DESOLATION WILDERNESS

FOREST

Cliff Lake

Jakes Peak

Rubicon Lake

N

0   0.5   1.0   1.5 miles

0   0.5   1.0   1.5 kilometers

Overview

The trail to Crag Lake may just whet the appetite of those who want to get past the crowds and set a bivy for a night under the stars. Rubicon fills the bill for solitude. Hike southwest along Meeks Creek, steadily ascending to Genevieve Lake and then Crag Lake. A side trip to Hidden Lake is not unwarranted for those who wish to be, well, hidden. But just a moderate climb past Shadow Lake and Stony Ridge Lake heads you up to the last 500 vertical feet to Rubicon Lake.

Route Details

The trail is cleverly signed TRAIL at the locked green gate. Duck under or go around the barrier, and walk nearly 1.5 miles on a dirt road, passing a long meadow, where you will see a marker indicating that your path is part of the Tahoe–Yosemite Trail. In another mile, as you come abreast of a small meadow, watch for the wilderness sign, a reminder that you need a permit.

Cross some good spots for filling your water bottles, including one crossing on a very stout footbridge, as you ascend Meeks Creek. The trail varies from soft duff to lumpy rock and dirt to tedious sand, along with granite stairs as you climb to petite Lake Genevieve. The General Creek Trail joins from the west near the north shore of this

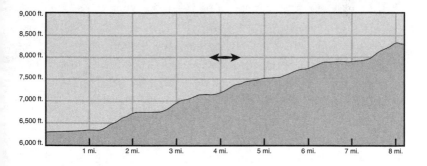

pretty tarn. Just 0.5 mile away is Crag Lake and its long shore, lined with red fir and Western white pine over some highly impacted sites that are good for picnics.

Leave Crag on a sand-and-rock trail, and watch your step as you look at the rock formations across the lake. Climb gently to the south and make a lazy switchback after crossing a stream on boulders. Then look for a faint trail leading to Hidden Lake. This lake makes for a nice diversion on the way home.

Ascend on a gentle, lodgepole-covered slope. Walk past the spur trail to Shadow Lake when you emerge from the trees. Keep above this pond, which is more like a flooded meadow, as the trail heads southeast. Within 20 minutes, you will arrive at long Stony Ridge Lake, stretched out beneath Rubicon Peak. A small trail at the north end of the lake crosses the outlet stream and leads to good bivy sites. The western shore has several picnic sites with a nice view of the lake.

The trail along Stony Ridge Lake provides a pleasant 0.6-mile amble with these superb views of Rubicon Peak tagging along. There are a few choice spots right along the trail where you can sit in the shade and relax in near solitude looking out on the lake. When you return to the trail, you'll soon be treated to bursts of trailside color.

Lupine and mountain ash crowd the base of lodgepole and juniper as the trail becomes somewhat marshy leaving Stony Ridge Lake. Look for surprising displays of Sierra lily along the spongy path. As the trail leads away from this long lake, causeways will help you across the wet areas. Soon it becomes crowded with sedges and small white flowers then passes under a huge wall of granite. Traverse the granite outcrop and cross another flower-bound stream—or butterfly magnet, if you will—where lupine, paintbrush, corn lily, daisy, aster, and bumblebees reside.

Immediately, then, you start the first leg of five long and three short switchbacks up to the rim of this next tarn. Granite steps are well placed along here to assist your vertical goal. Just before you reach the lake, turn around and capture the vista back down onto

Stony Ridge Lake. Cross the granite, and your sand-and-duff trail leads up and over to a point with a whole-lake vista.

Some highly impacted campsites are adjacent to the lake just below the trail. They are well concealed and on a durable surface, but unfortunately they are right on top of the lake. Find better bivy sites by following the trail past the lakeside boulders and granite to the saddle overlooking both Rubicon and Grouse Lakes. There is also a bivy site among the boulders at the north end of the lake that may keep you out of the wind. Enjoy the stars here, and follow the trail downhill *mañana*.

Directions

The Meeks Creek Trailhead is 11.5 miles south of Tahoe City on CA 89. The trailhead parking lot is on the west side of the road, across from Meeks Bay Campground and Marina. Park in the small dirt lot, which has room for about 10 cars. There are no facilities here. Additional parking can be found along the highway.

34 Barker Pass to Echo Lakes

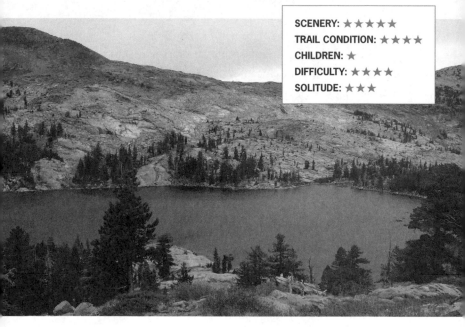

SCENERY: ★ ★ ★ ★ ★
TRAIL CONDITION: ★ ★ ★
CHILDREN: ★
DIFFICULTY: ★ ★ ★ ★
SOLITUDE: ★ ★ ★

OFTEN WINDBLOWN, DICKS LAKE HAS SOME SHELTERED CAMPSITES.

GPS TRAILHEAD COORDINATES: N39° 04.594′ W120° 14.101′ (Barker Pass),
N38° 50.118′ W120° 02.654′ (Echo Lakes)

DISTANCE & CONFIGURATION: 33-mile point-to-point with shuttle

HIKING TIME: 2 nights

OUTSTANDING FEATURES: Visit eight sparkling lakes, traverse wildflower-filled meadows,
and enjoy expansive vistas of the Desolation Wilderness and the Crystal Range.

ELEVATION: 7,650′ at trailhead

ACCESS: Depends on snow. This hike enters the Desolation Wilderness at Lost Corner
Mountain and so requires a wilderness permit stating the location of your first night's
camp. Overnight camping permits are available for a fee at US Forest Service or Lake
Tahoe Basin Management Unit visitor centers, or online at tinyurl.com/dwovernightcamping.

MAPS: *Tahoe Rim Trail* (Tom Harrison Maps)

FACILITIES: Pit toilet

CONTACT: US Forest Service, Lake Tahoe Basin Management Unit, 530-543-2600,
www.fs.usda.gov/ltbmu

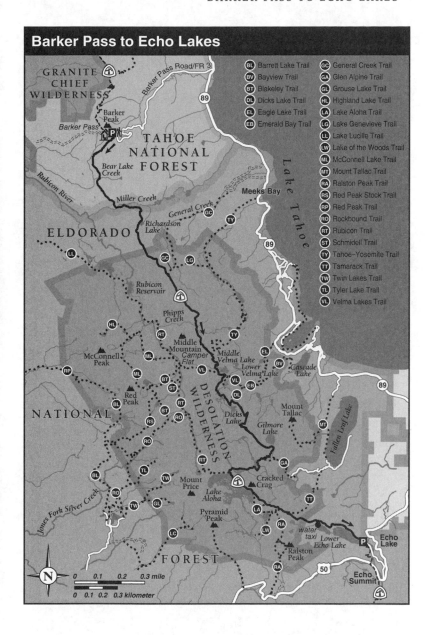

Barker Pass to Echo Lakes

BL	Barrett Lake Trail	**GC**	General Creek Trail
BV	Bayview Trail	**GA**	Glen Alpine Trail
BT	Blakeley Trail	**GL**	Grouse Lake Trail
DL	Dicks Lake Trail	**HL**	Highland Lake Trail
EL	Eagle Lake Trail	**LA**	Lake Aloha Trail
EB	Emerald Bay Trail	**LG**	Lake Genevieve Trail
		LL	Lake Lucille Trail
		LW	Lake of the Woods Trail
		ML	McConnell Lake Trail
		MT	Mount Tallac Trail
		RA	Ralston Peak Trail
		RS	Red Peak Stock Trail
		RP	Red Peak Trail
		RO	Rockbound Trail
		RT	Rubicon Trail
		ST	Schmidell Trail
		TY	Tahoe–Yosemite Trail
		TT	Tamarack Trail
		TW	Twin Lakes Trail
		TL	Tyler Lake Trail
		VL	Velma Lakes Trail

Overview

Immerse yourself in the Desolation Wilderness, or at least in one of the eight mountain lakes that you visit on this three-day adventure. You will tread on both the Tahoe Rim Trail (TRT) and the Pacific Crest Trail (PCT), as they follow the same track on this hike. The first day is the longest yet is still a moderate hike of 15 miles and about 1,000 up-and-down feet, to placid Middle Velma Lake. Day two starts with a brief climb to Fontanillis and Dicks Lakes and then begins a switchbacking climb to cross Dicks Pass. One word: *vistas*. Descend and pass more liquid gems, dazzlingly bright in the light reflected from the surrounding granite. Camp near Lake Aloha and enjoy an easy day's hike along its shore, passing three more lakes on your way downhill to Echo Lakes.

Route Details

Use the picnic table under the trees at the trailhead to recheck and reassemble your gear as well as to affix your permit to your backpack. (Rangers will check for permits, and they *will* escort unpermitted hikers out via the closest trailhead.) If you need a map, stop at the trailhead kiosk and pick up one of the "green maps" provided for your safety by the Tahoe Rim Trail Association. This section of the TRT coincides with the PCT, so the grade and track are mellow and well maintained.

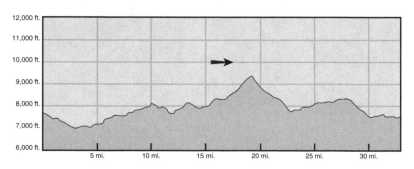

Dropping off the road like a skater into a bowl, you begin by circumnavigating the open mouth of the basin, called Cothrin Cove. If only the trail could traverse the upper rim of this snow bowl, then the trail would be a straight line south. Alas, the PCT strives to maintain an average trail grade below 10%, and so a beeline would ruin the average (and cause a lot of grumbling). So around the horns of this dilemma you go, about 6 miles to Richardson Lake, nestled at the foot of Sourdough Hill. Your track descends about 650 feet and then regains about 450 feet to reach Richardson.

All of the elevation gain will be fully appreciated, for over the next few miles the vistas of Rockbound Valley are stunning. View Rubicon Reservoir, Rockbound Lake, Buck Island Lake, and the Rubicon River as it builds coming down this lithic trench.

Your trail to the Velma Lakes area is like a roller coaster at a small summer carnival—some up, some down, and some turns but no surprises and nothing frightening. From Richardson, ascend 650 feet over 4 miles, and then descend 400 feet in 2 miles. Reclaim that height in the next 1.4 miles, then lose 250 and gain 50 getting to Middle Velma Lake. Now it's cotton candy time. Look around at the choice of campsites visible above Middle Velma. To remain on the PCT/TRT pathway, this lake is your choice. If you don't mind straying off this described route, you have other options for your bivy site. For a more detailed description of the route to this point, see the next hike, Barker Pass to Middle Velma Lake.

Middle Velma has easy access from two popular trailheads, so it invites small crowds of day hikers to its shores. Although I have not had feet on the ground there, Lower Velma can be reached by descending Upper Velma's outlet creek about 150 feet to the granite shores, where it appears that there is some solitude to be gained. There are other sites at Upper Velma and its unnamed companion as well. So, depending on where you set your camp, alternate routes will still keep you ultimately on track.

If the south shore of Middle Velma is arrayed with tents and you don't want to lose elevation going to the lower lake, walk to the junction at the southeast corner of the lake. This hike follows the trail south to Fontanillis Lake and then east to Dicks Lake and over Dicks Pass. To camp in the vicinity of Upper Velma, walk about 200 yards east, following the marker to the Bayview Trail. The next junction marks a trail to your right that leads to Upper Velma Lake. The trail rounds the lake, crossing the inlet at its south end, and then follows the base of the moraine that parallels Fontanillis.

If you want to proceed from the Upper Velma–Bayview junction another 250 yards to explore campsites around the unnamed lake, be assured that you have another alternate route that will not let you miss Dicks Pass. Now on the Bayview Trail, heading east, a large log will help you cross the outlet stream, which has widened into a small pond here. The marshy end of this lake will soon come into view on your right. You can exit the trail as you head around the easternmost node of the lake. Juniper, white pine, lodgepole, and fir are scattered around this secluded lake.

To resume your hike from this unnamed lake, you could always return to the Fontanillis–Bayview junction and continue on the PCT. Or you can continue east on the Bayview Trail to the junction with the trail to Dicks Lake at about 8,240 feet in elevation. As you hike to that body of water, you will pass the intersection of the trail coming around the south end of Upper Velma; 0.25 mile past that point is the junction with the PCT/TRT heading south across Dicks Pass.

But if you take either of those alternates, you'll miss two spectacular lakes and some wonderful vistas. So leave the Velma Lakes area by way of the trail leading to Fontanillis Lake. The uphill grind is abated by the pleasant shade of red fir and lodgepole pine above the mellow switchbacks.

Fontanillis sports no more than a few dozen trees, mostly at the north end, where one could siesta but not camp. The trail requires watching as you cross the outlet stream heading into Upper Velma. But before you continue across the channel, stop for a photo of the terrain and lakes spread before you, all the way to Lake Tahoe. Granite reaching out from the flanks of Dicks Peak both intrudes on and encloses Fontanillis's waters. The trail skirts the boggy boulder field around the lake, then heads away on a southeast bearing toward Dicks Lake. A scant half-mile of rocky trail leads you to Dicks Lake, where a junction marker points you north on the trail for Dicks Pass. So take a left unless you need to filter water, which you could easily do 200 feet over at the lake.

Don't be alarmed by heading northwest away from the lake, as you'll hit another junction to Dicks Pass in barely 0.25 mile. This rocky saddle offers a vista onto Lake Tahoe before turning away to the east to begin your zigzag ascent. Views onto the lake from the shaded trail are more awesome with each small elevation gain. The switchbacks are fairly easy and not steep; even so, wooden stairs assist at the hardest spots.

Reaching the open saddle at Dicks Pass, you have vistas to Castle Peak and Sierra Buttes. The sandy trail across the pass heads through hemlocks that have been windswept and stunted. This is a great place to take a break; with vistas and sunshine all around, you can look down on Half Moon and Alta Morris Lakes, off to Susie Lake, out to Lake Aloha with Pyramid Peak and Mount Price visible beyond it, and over to Dicks Peak much closer at hand.

The next 2.3 miles see your trail dropping about 1,000 feet to the shores of Gilmore Lake. Begin descending from the pass on rocky trail on this scree-covered slope, where switchbacks lead you through hemlock and willow to small, colorful meadows. On this wet, south-facing slope, you will see yellow monkeyflower, fireweed, gentian, paintbrush, asters, and yarrow as you find a spot to relax overlooking Half Moon Lake. Level out under the scattered lodgepole pines as you approach Gilmore Lake from the south. Nathan Gilmore discovered the mineral waters at Glen Alpine Springs, and he also pastured his sheep and Angora goats in this area. With easy access to filter water and take a dip, this is a fine spot for taking lunch.

Retreat from Gilmore by heading south on the trail leading to Glen Alpine, loosely following the outlet stream from this round lake. A couple of junctions ahead will cause some head-scratching, but that's why you have a map. At the first marked junction, at the bottom of the stairs, a trail leads acutely to the right and heads to Half Moon Lake. About 25 feet away, the Glen Alpine Trail goes left where your trail to Lake Aloha heads right.

When you reach the next marker about 200 feet below you, it may seem like déjà vu, but just follow the marker's arrow to the right for Aloha, Susie, and Heather Lakes. Cross the double stream here on the ample boulders provided, and begin ascending the moraine on Susie Lake's east side. You have to walk around this watery obstacle to get to the trail's exit point just behind the islands. The trail stays above the shore level until after crossing the lake's outlet. You'll spot many shaded spots along the heather-lined shore that are appropriate for filtering water or having a siesta, but they are too close for camping. Round the lake's southern shore, and the trail will slide by the island-bearing cove just before heading uphill toward Heather Lake.

A brief climb of less than 150 feet will take you to a traverse under steep slopes to Heather Lake. Approach the lake at the mouth, where a blaze has been long ago carved into the lodgepole standing sentinel here. You won't be faulted for looking up twice to the right just to make sure all that talus stays in place. (Don't wiggle that "one" rock.) Ringed by solid and decaying granite, Heather Lake is graced with trees only at its inlets. There's no good camping near Heather, but there are excellent sites on the rock well above its western shore. The ever-popular granite stairs help you ascend the 250 feet to overlook Lake Aloha. The trail to Mosquito Pass traverses the northern shore of Aloha and leads across the pass to Clyde Lake and Rockbound Valley.

This area above the lake but below the trail can offer some private bivy spots, but finding shelter from the wind is another matter. Good bivy sites are available on the granite slopes east of the PCT as it parallels the lake. Waking up just as the sun just strikes the peaks that tower over Aloha—Pyramid, Agassiz, and Price—is a memorable moment. Day three begins by roughly paralleling Aloha's shore on a rocky trail.

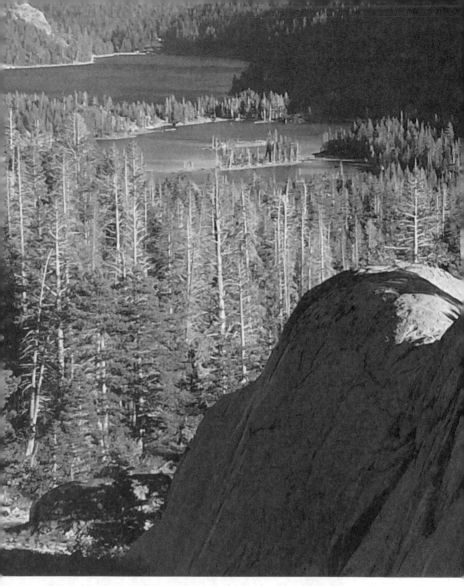

THE ECHO LAKES COME INTO VIEW AS YOU DESCEND FROM ALOHA.

As you walk beneath Cracked Crag along the rock-lined path to the southeast, you may realize how the permit fees that you paid actually impact the wilderness. Of the many trail junctions, stream crossings, and steep slopes that the PCT and TRT encounter, I have found only one unmarked junction, and that is near the end of Lake

Aloha. Immediately after entering trees, look for a junction marked by a blank post. Do not continue along in the trees bordering the lake. Rather, turn uphill on the obvious angled path that leads to Lakes Lucille and Margery. (Continuing straight would have taken you slightly out of the way to Lake of the Woods. Many paths intersect in this area, so a mistake in navigation is understandable and not too difficult to recover from.)

This long, gently sloping path is a pleasant section of trail. Several junctions over the course of the next 0.5 mile offer tempting destinations, but you can just keep going straight toward Echo Lakes. Pass the trails to Lucille, Margery, Aloha, and Lake of the Woods, catching an occasional glimpse of Mount Tallac to the north. This traverse offers you time to slow down, not work so hard, and enjoy the flowers that foretell the upcoming Haypress Meadows. Skirt the top of the meadow just after passing the last Aloha trail, then pass through a copse of conifers surrounding the path to Lake of the Woods.

Cross the meadow and begin a gentle descent, bypassing the left-hand junction of the trail leading across the slope to Triangle Lake. The PCT/TRT now begins descending in earnest, beginning with a well-placed pair of switchbacks. Your views of Tamarack, Cagwin, and Ralston Lakes and their surrounding peaks do nothing but improve over the next half-mile. Your superb vista onto Tamarack is eclipsed by a down-canyon view to the east of Upper and Lower Echo Lakes. After all cameras are stowed, cross a stone bridge to enter a stand of lodgepole on a dirt-and-duff trail.

Your continued descent crosses more stoneworks and passes another link to Triangle Lake before exiting the Desolation Wilderness. As you approach the north end of Upper Echo Lake, you can leave the exposed rock and enjoy the shade of tall lodgepole, to which early settlers mistakenly ascribed the appellation of tamarack. Attached to one of these, high above the trail, is a small marker signaling the trail down to the small dock and a phone for the Echo Lakes water taxi. This is an easily missed trail, so watch for it if you really want to spring for the $12 fare to save a 3-mile hike. (There is a $36 minimum as well. Still, it's a nice hike.)

Stone culverts contain some of the several runoff streams that sneak down from the left. As you traverse east for the next 0.6 mile, the tread remains about 300 feet from the shore and about 100 feet above it. Reaching a high point above the channel separating upper from lower, the trail turns to give a view of Flagpole Peak above Lower Echo. The PCT stays above a local path useful only to the cabin owners below. Pass an intersection that leads down to these cabins, and stay on the higher trail.

When the trail ascends about as high above lake level as it is going to, your granite path becomes narrower but still safe. In fact, you can see that the safety railings have long ago been cut away. This is a dicey spot during winter travel. About 0.25 mile ahead, almost directly underneath Flagpole Peak, is another pair of descending switchbacks followed by an innocuous junction with the lower trail to the cabins. With the thought of having a cold milk shake at the Echo Lake Chalet firmly in your mind, the last mile to the lake's outlet should be even easier along this level granite-and-sand path.

Before descending to the lake level, continue ahead to the obvious vista point looking out to Lake Tahoe in the north and Freel Peak in the east. Walk downhill, bypassing any turns until you reach the bottom, where the trail passes the TRT kiosk on the right. Follow the shaded path to the outlet, where you can cross on an open metal walkway and concrete dam. The chalet is on the left, and cold drinks are served there daily. To reach Echo Summit, follow the PCT/TRT signs for the pathway near the pit toilets leading up to the parking area.

Directions

Starting in Tahoe City, drive south on CA 89 for 4.2 miles to Blackwood Canyon Road. Marked with signs for a snow park and the Kaspian Campground, this turn is 0.6 mile north of Tahoe Pines and 22.9 miles from South Lake Tahoe.

Turn west and drive 2.3 miles. Jog to the left, where Forest Road 15N38 continues straight ahead. Drive across the bridge spanning Blackwood Creek and jog to the right, then drive 4.7 miles southwest up Barker Pass Road/FR 3. The trailhead parking is ahead on the right, about 0.5 mile after the pavement ends.

There is a small parking lot with room for about a dozen cars, a pit toilet, and a TRT information kiosk with maps, but no trash receptacles. Two picnic tables and a decent area for tents are adjacent for PCT hikers to crash and prepare their packs.

The signed trailhead is across the road from the end of the parking lot driveway.

You'll also need to leave a shuttle vehicle at Echo Summit. From South Lake Tahoe, drive 4.8 miles south on US 50 to Meyers. Stay on US 50 past CA 89 for 5 more miles, then turn right onto Johnson Pass Road. This is a sharp right turn off of a long bend around Echo Summit, so here are some checkpoints: There is a Caltrans maintenance station at the tip of the bend (3.8 miles from Meyers). Your turn is a sharp right 1.2 miles ahead, just past the renovation-ready Little Norway.

To reach Echo Summit from Placerville, drive 39.8 miles to Strawberry. Johnson Pass Road is on the left, 7.4 miles past Strawberry and 1.8 miles past Sierra-at-Tahoe ski resort. Follow the angled road as above. Drive 0.6 mile along Johnson Pass Road to a left turn onto Echo Lakes Road, and stay left 0.9 mile until you reach the large parking lot above the Echo Lakes Chalet. You can unload packs but not park down below in front of the chalet, but it's pretty easy to park up top and take the trail and steps leading from the north side of the lot down through the trees, behind the pit toilets, to the chalet.

35

Barker Pass to Middle Velma Lake

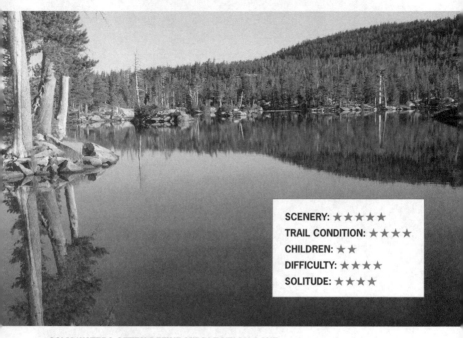

SCENERY: ★★★★★
TRAIL CONDITION: ★★★★
CHILDREN: ★★
DIFFICULTY: ★★★★
SOLITUDE: ★★★★

CALM WATERS OFTEN DEFINE MIDDLE VELMA LAKE.

GPS TRAILHEAD COORDINATES: N39° 04.594′ W120° 14.101′

DISTANCE & CONFIGURATION: 30.2-mile out-and-back

HIKING TIME: 18 hours (overnight)

OUTSTANDING FEATURES: Hike along the Pacific Crest Trail, the Tahoe Rim Trail, and the Tahoe–Yosemite Trail as they all lead to one of the most beautiful lakes in the Desolation Wilderness.

ELEVATION: 7,650′ at trailhead

ACCESS: Depends on snow. You´ll be hiking and camping overnight in the Desolation Wilderness, so you´ll need a permit, available at the Taylor Creek Visitor Center or online at tinyurl.com/dwovernightcamping.

MAPS: *Tahoe Rim Trail* (Tom Harrison Maps)

FACILITIES: Pit toilet

CONTACT: US Forest Service, Lake Tahoe Basin Management Unit, 530-543-2600, www.fs.usda.gov/ltbmu

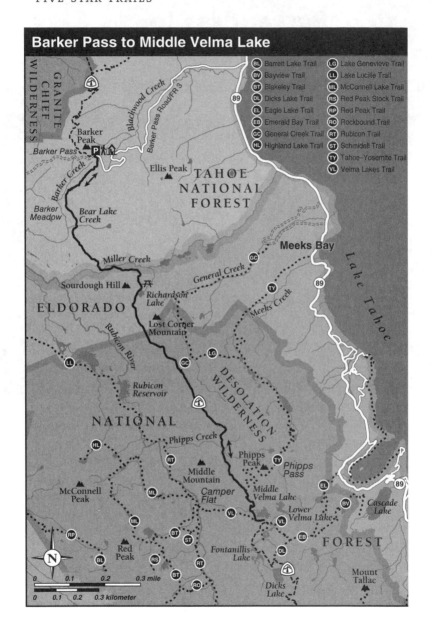

Barker Pass to Middle Velma Lake

BL Barrett Lake Trail	**LG** Lake Genevieve Trail
BV Bayview Trail	**LL** Lake Lucille Trail
BT Blakeley Trail	**ML** McConnell Lake Trail
DL Dicks Lake Trail	**RS** Red Peak Stock Trail
EL Eagle Lake Trail	**RP** Red Peak Trail
EB Emerald Bay Trail	**RO** Rockbound Trail
GC General Creek Trail	**RT** Rubicon Trail
HL Highland Lake Trail	**ST** Schmidell Trail
	TY Tahoe–Yosemite Trail
	VL Velma Lakes Trail

Overview

Velma Lakes are popular on summer weekends because they are close to Eagle Falls and the trail from Eagle Lake, but if you have a chance to arrive midweek, you may have the waters to yourself. The trail is a long roller coaster through forest and rock with plenty of streams, springs, lakes, and meadows decorated with wildflowers. Navigation is easy on this southbound trek, as you never leave the Pacific Crest Trail (PCT) and there are relatively few distracting junctions.

Route Details

Pick up a map provided by the Tahoe Rim Trail Association at the kiosk, tighten your buckles, and step off the edge of dusty Barker Pass Road. Head downhill across the first meadow, where a few springs provoke a word of thanks for Gore-Tex. Larkspur, paintbrush, columbine, and elderberry are prolific in the meadows along this downhill traverse. Turn southwest at another small meadow, and reenter the forest for a moment until you cross another small meadow. The bright-green, mosslike plant adorning the trees is wolf lichen, and it grows readily on red firs.

Pass by Barker Meadow just before you come abreast of Barker Creek and, shortly, Bear Lake Road. Stay nearly parallel to it for about

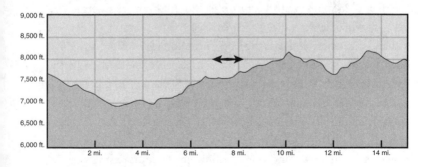

0.5 mile as you curve around the northern horn of the basin called Cothrin Cove, below Bear Lake. Cross this same off-highway vehicle (OHV) track after about 2.4 miles from the trailhead. A quick jog left and jag right picks up the trail leading to a crossing of Bear Lake's outlet 0.4 mile ahead.

The dirt-and-duff trail continues around the southern horn, heading about 1.5 miles to a crossing of the Rubicon–McKinney OHV Road, which leads down to Tahoma. It is, according to the sign but disputed by some, 4 miles back to Barker Pass (let's call that between 4 and 4.5) and 9 miles to Twin Peaks. Go straight across the road, and follow an easterly course on the sandy trail bordered by boulders. Head southeast 675 feet to a crossing of Miller Creek, where you will find acceptable bivy spots to the left on the west side of the creek.

Traverse slightly uphill as you head east, navigating around Sourdough Hill. The trees block any view of it or of Miller Meadows, about 200 yards from the trail. Climb to the south around and over the feet of Sourdough Hill on the way to a lunchtime break at compact Richardson Lake, about 0.5 mile after the trail turns south away from Miller Creek. Richardson Lake is accessible by off-highway vehicles, and the impact here shows heavy traffic but respectful practices.

Depart your poolside café, and traverse southwest along the side of Sourdough again. Cross the OHV road at the signpost in the middle of the saddle, and begin an uphill traverse, gaining about 425 feet over the next 3.25 miles. With Lost Corner Mountain on your left shoulder, you will start to notice good vistas of the Desolation Wilderness just about the time you pass the wilderness boundary. Enjoy the views down to Rockbound Lake and Rubicon Reservoir and then to the Crystal Range from Tells and McConnell to Silver and Red Peaks.

The General Creek Trail intersects this track about 9.9 miles from the trailhead. The sharp left turn to the north follows the creek and will lead hikers down to Ed Z'berg Sugar Pine Point State Park. However, your ascending trail steadily heads southeast about 2.4 miles and then turns more directly south for a half-mile walk to the Phipps Creek crossing. The duff trail descends past a couple of small

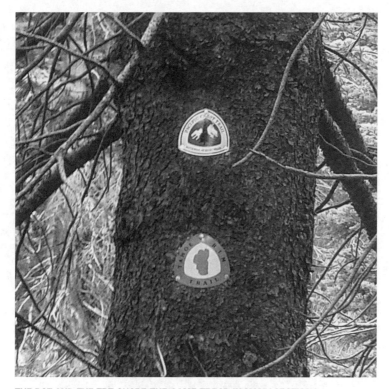

THE PCT AND THE TRT SHARE THE SAME TREAD IN MANY SECTIONS.

meadows and brings you to a fairly direct crossing of Phipps Creek followed by a brief, rocky uphill. Then you'll begin an easy southward traverse beneath red fir and lodgepole pine.

The Phipps Peak Trail joins your route just 1.6 miles after you cross Phipps Creek. Turning west here joins a trail skirting the southern flank of Phipps Peak and continuing across Phipps Pass before dropping to Rubicon, Stony Ridge, Crag, and Genevieve Lakes and on to the trailhead at Meeks Creek. This would make a good route for a shuttle trip day hike. However, the described trail continues about 1.5 miles farther to Middle Velma Lake.

Phipps Peak stands above your hat brim as you head southeast on this forested trail. Huge granite boulders crowd the stream crossing ahead. Follow the winding PCT, going south about where a causeway 0.85 mile from the junction assists you across a marshy area with gray, standing snags piercing the blue sky.

Briefly pass the west end of the lake as you head south. Be alert for the signed trail junction leading west to Camper Flat and Lake Schmidell. Turn east and head up above the south shore of the lake. Here you'll find several sites to set up your tent or bivy. As tempting as it is, the lakeside areas are highly impacted and generally not sanctioned as campsites. The granite slopes above the shore offer excellent choices for flat, dry spots.

Return the way you came after a couple of days of midweek solitude. If you have a shuttle car, an alternate exit is to take the Velma Lakes Trail 1 mile southeast and 0.7 mile east to a junction with the Eagle Lake Trail and the Bayview Trail. Depending on where you want to leave a shuttle, either route offers an excellent departure from the wilderness.

Directions

Starting in Tahoe City, drive south on CA 89 for 4.2 miles to Blackwood Canyon Road. Marked with signs for a snow park and the Kaspian Campground, this turn is 0.6 mile north of Tahoe Pines and 22.9 miles from South Lake Tahoe.

Drive 2.3 miles west, and jog left where Forest Road 15N38 continues straight ahead. Drive across the bridge spanning Blackwood Creek and jog right, then drive 4.7 miles southwest up Barker Pass Road/FR 3. The trailhead parking is ahead on the right, about 0.5 mile after the pavement ends.

There is a small parking lot with room for about a dozen cars, a pit toilet, and a Tahoe Rim Trail information kiosk with maps, but no trash receptacles. PCT hikers can fiddle with their packs at the two picnic tables near a semidecent area for tents.

The signed trailhead is across the road from the end of the parking lot driveway.

36

Barker Pass
to Twin Peaks

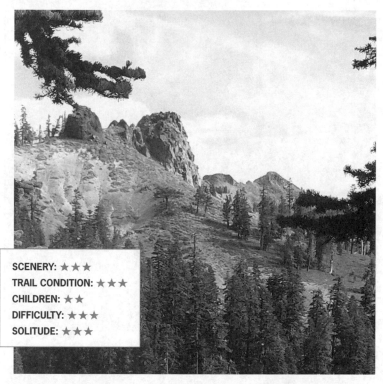

AT TWIN PEAKS, VIEWS MAY INCLUDE THE LAKE OR VOLCANIC DEBRIS.

SCENERY: ★★★
TRAIL CONDITION: ★★★
CHILDREN: ★★
DIFFICULTY: ★★★
SOLITUDE: ★★★

GPS TRAILHEAD COORDINATES: N39° 04.624′ W120° 14.110′

DISTANCE & CONFIGURATION: 11.4-mile out-and-back

HIKING TIME: 6 hours

OUTSTANDING FEATURES: Outstanding vistas of Lake Tahoe, Desolation Wilderness, and Granite Chief Wilderness; wildflower-covered meadows fed by the many runoff streams

ELEVATION: 7,680′ at trailhead

ACCESS: Depends on snow

MAPS: *Lake Tahoe Basin* (Trails Illustrated 803)

FACILITIES: Pit toilet

CONTACT: US Forest Service, Lake Tahoe Basin Management Unit, 530-543-2600, www.fs.usda.gov/ltbmu

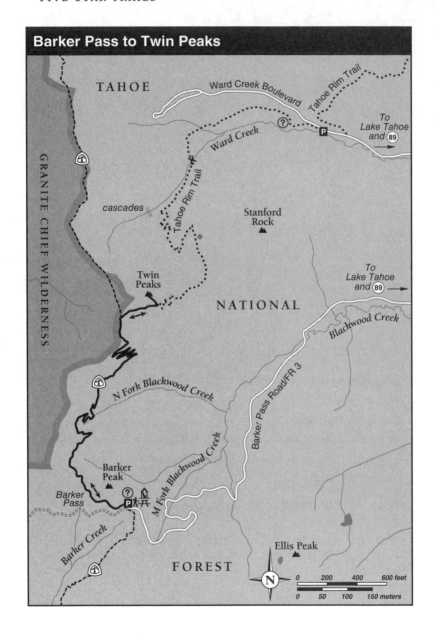

Barker Pass to Twin Peaks

Overview

This hike follows the Pacific Crest Trail (PCT) and Tahoe Rim Trail (TRT) until they diverge near your destination. It has its ups and downs, literally. For about the first 1.5 miles from the trailhead, gain 600 feet, then lose 475 feet of it over an equivalent distance, only to repeat the first process with another zigzagging 750-foot climb over about 2.3 miles to approach the summit. Then another 200 feet of vertical travel over 500 feet will hoist you to the summit, where the views all around are incredible.

Route Details

After you've re-sorted your gear and snacked at the picnic table, read the interpretive display, picked up a TRT map, and visited the pit toilet, it's time to hit the trail heading west. Start out overlooking Barker Creek Basin as you head around to the northwest, circling the peak named after a local pioneering rancher.

After 0.8 mile, one stream crossing, and one logging-road crossing, get your camera ready for a beautiful vista east toward Lake Tahoe, looking down the tree-filled trough called Blackwood Canyon. Fair campsites can be found nearby, where a social trail intersects the PCT/TRT.

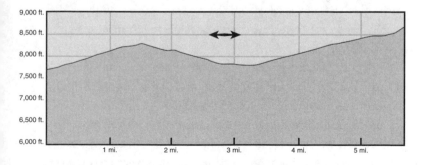

Climb to a tiny meadow on a dirt trail leading to a three-section causeway across the wettest area of this flower magnet. Indian paintbrush, corn lily, and lupine color the ground here as the flowers just flow downhill. The dirt trail soon turns to rock as you climb across a lightly treed scree slope. After 1.5 miles, you have a great view onto the lake from right in the middle of this rockfest. The path heads toward a knob of red volcanic scoria and rock. Follow the trail sign to pass to the west of this knob.

Checkerspot butterflies may escort you down the trail along long switchbacks down into and across a ravine. Runoff streams are plentiful in this large, glacially excavated sluice. Fireweed and larkspur decorate the trail at every wet crossing as you descend and recross the meadow on a couple of long, loopy switchbacks. Near the bottom of the meadow, around 2.3 miles in, you come skidding to a halt next to the steep-sided ravine containing the North Fork Blackwood Creek. The volcanic geology is impressive here.

Contour north across a steep slope, stepping across three more runoff streams pouring down from the walls of rock above the trail. As you take switchbacks down, vistas of Tahoe continue to tempt photographers.

Contour along without much effort on this duff trail beneath the cover of cone-laden firs for the next 0.5 mile. Cross a rockfall on a steep slope, and then ascend a bit to the first of six switchbacks. You get another view of the lake from this first turn. These gently graded switchbacks weave across the slope, staying in the shade of firs up to near the ridge.

Round the corner coming over a ridge of an unnamed peak to once again spy your uphill destination. Traverse the north-facing slope, and your dirt trail crosses the boundary of the Granite Chief Wilderness at 4.75 miles along. Who has the permit? Within a few hundred feet, you'll have another photo opportunity. Follow along as the trail traverses this exposed ridgetop with its vistas to the west. Enter the cover of firs again before the PCT and TRT diverge in 0.2

mile. Keep to the right at the signed trail junction at 5.5 miles, and head uphill with the dual summits over your left shoulder.

Pass beneath the debris of these two pointed monoliths—summit dandruff—for the next 0.5 mile. The summit trail's junction with the TRT is at the southeastern ridge of the hill. The TRT continues immediately downhill on tight switchbacks while the summit trail turns left, northwest, through tobacco brush and climbs across the manzanita-speckled slope to the ridge. Walk steeply up along the edge of the drop-off until the obvious trail disappears.

To gain either summit requires Class 3 climbing skills—basically using hands and feet along with good balance. To reach the east summit, cross to the west through the fir trees. Leave the ridge and head to the talus-and-boulder rockfall below the summit. No trail marks the final ascent to the summit. Serpentine across the rock pile to make your way up. Vistas reach out to Dicks Peak in the Desolation Wilderness and Ward's Peak, Granite Chief, and Squaw Peak as well as the blue water of Lake Tahoe below Homewood across to Freel Peak at the southeast corner of the lake.

Directions

Starting in Tahoe City, drive south on CA 89 for 4.2 miles to Blackwood Canyon Road. Marked with signs for a snow park and the Kaspian Picnic Area, this turn is 0.6 mile north of Tahoe Pines and 22.9 miles from South Lake Tahoe.

Drive 2.3 miles west, and jog left where Forest Road 15N38 continues straight ahead. Drive across the bridge spanning Blackwood Creek, and jog right, and then drive 4.7 miles southwest up Barker Pass Road/FR 3. The trailhead is ahead on the right, about 0.5 mile after the pavement ends.

The trailhead is adjacent to a small parking lot with room for about a dozen cars. There is a pit toilet and a TRT information kiosk with maps, but no trash receptacles. Two picnic tables are handy for hikers making last-minute gear adjustments.

Ward Creek to Twin Peaks

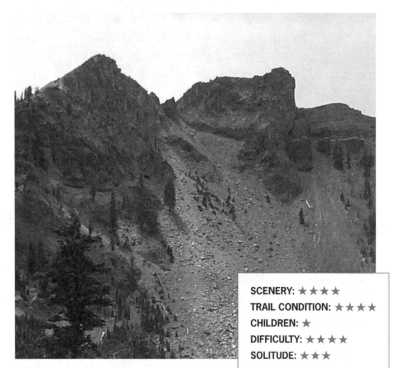

SCENERY: ★ ★ ★ ★
TRAIL CONDITION: ★ ★ ★ ★
CHILDREN: ★
DIFFICULTY: ★ ★ ★ ★
SOLITUDE: ★ ★

DEFINITELY NOT THE SIDE TO ASCEND

GPS TRAILHEAD COORDINATES: N39° 08.428′ W120° 11.507′

DISTANCE & CONFIGURATION: 12-mile out-and-back

HIKING TIME: 5–6 hours

OUTSTANDING FEATURES: 360-degree vistas of Granite Chief Wilderness and Lake Tahoe; relatively moderate hiking; meadow after meadow of flowers

ELEVATION: 6,550′ at trailhead

ACCESS: Depends on snow

MAPS: *Lake Tahoe Basin* (Trails Illustrated 803)

FACILITIES: None

CONTACT: US Forest Service, Lake Tahoe Basin Management Unit, 530-543-2600, www.fs.usda.gov/ltbmu

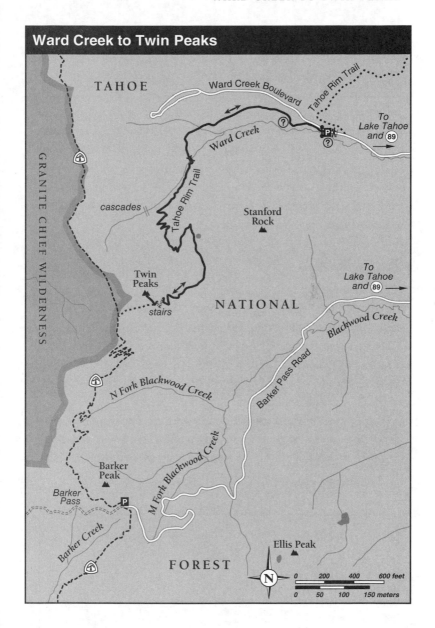

Ward Creek to Twin Peaks

Overview

This brief segment of the Tahoe Rim Trail (TRT) climbs to the margin of the Granite Chief Wilderness and sneaks breathtaking views of it and Lake Tahoe from above Tahoe Pines and Homewood. A leisurely walk up the old road leads to a trail that continues up Ward Creek Canyon. Cross it and stay above its east bank before leaving it on switchbacks. Approaching the peaks from this direction gives a new perspective on this pair of rocks. Climb to the rim of the forested cirque, and navigate around it to the easternmost horn of rock. A Class 3 scramble leads to excellent vistas past Barker Peak to the south and north across Ward Peak.

Route Details

This section of the TRT leads back to Tahoe City or forward, joining the Pacific Crest Trail (PCT) on the west side of Twin Peaks. Pick up a green map, and walk past the locked gate on the dirt-and-gravel road. About 200 feet along is a kiosk with information regarding the Ward Creek riparian zone and stream habitat. Another similar kiosk stands 0.4 mile ahead.

The road passes through a lodgepole–Jeffrey pine forest about 1.8 miles and sideswipes a dirt mound where you might spot a marker for Twin Peaks to the right where the tread has been rerouted. Cross a stream immediately after this reassuring signpost. A half-mile from

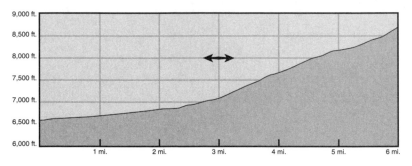

here, your crossing of Ward Creek will be via footbridge. Just before reaching the bridge, step across another small stream. The bridge is marked with a plaque on the north side. The south side has but a path down to the creek.

A direction change to the southwest leads you past a small meadow as you begin to parallel the creek. Although unseen through the trees, the frogs and birds along the stream make their presence known to hikers. Woolly mule's ears populate the next small meadow, which is made all the more special by its fringe of aspens adding music to the air. Continue southwest among the fir trees.

Cross a couple of streams as you traverse 0.8 mile from the bridge to the first switchback. Enter the cirque, and the trail turns away from the creek, beginning to gain meaningful elevation. Look for a small waterfall that can be seen from the stone stairs at the end of the second switchback. Above that, the rocky trail crosses a sloped meadow thick with mule's ears, aster, and lupine. The trail enters and exits the same meadow at each higher switchback. The flower displays repeat at every turn on this ride.

Now, at about 7,300 feet and with your destination in sight, head toward it, and then turn on a long, circuitous path away from it. Continue climbing south briefly, and begin a swing around to the east followed by a lazy turn to the north, climbing across one meadow after another. These meadows all seem to be fed by a spring next to the trail on the next southeast leg, which carries you about 0.5 mile to the ridge and a junction with the trail on the left leading to Stanford Rock and on to Ward Creek State Park. This point is about 5 miles away from the trailhead and about a mile to the peak.

Follow the outline of the cirque, stopping along the way to take pictures to the north and into the maw of this glacial remnant. About 500 feet shy of the summit, the Western hemlocks become so thick that the trail at noon seems completely shaded. That is, however, a real comfort as the trail climbs and switches back across the slope. Some stone stairs help you up through a particularly steep section of the forest just before you reach a brief plateau.

The TRT separates from this route just about 300 feet beneath the summit, then continues to the left to join the PCT southward. Your obvious route climbs to the right through the tobacco brush and manzanita and across the rocky slope littered with random mule's ears. Just after you pass the fallen white pine, Lake Tahoe appears above the trees. Fir and hemlock crowd the way as you edge closer to the north, right up to the rim. The dirt trail climbs a bit on this edge, and when it reaches the largest hemlock, you veer left to the talus rockfall beneath the summit. Cross the talus to the west, and then work back up to the east to gain the windy summit. Pictures taken, this is not a summit for relaxing on, so retreat the way you entered.

Directions

From South Lake Tahoe, drive 24.8 miles north on CA 89 to Pineland Drive on the left. Signs on the highway for an RV village are a large landmark. Turn left (west) on Pineland, which will in 0.4 mile turn into Ward Creek Boulevard. Park in any small pullout on the left, 2.2 miles from the highway. The pullouts are hard to see, so watch your odometer closely.

Pineland Drive is 2.3 miles south of Tahoe City. Turn right (west) on Pineland and drive 2.2 miles. The trailhead is just off the road, at the Tahoe Rim Trail marker and informational kiosk. Pick up a map here before embarking.

There are no facilities at this trailhead.

38

Mount Judah Loop

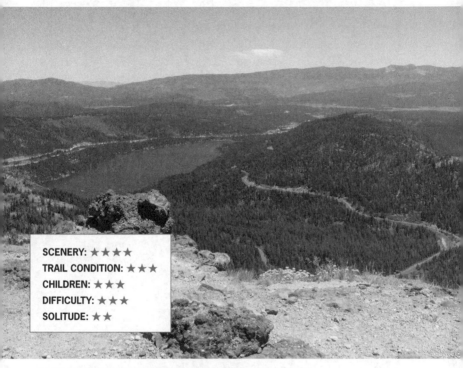

SCENERY: ★ ★ ★ ★
TRAIL CONDITION: ★ ★ ★
CHILDREN: ★ ★ ★
DIFFICULTY: ★ ★ ★
SOLITUDE: ★ ★

MOUNT JUDAH OFFERS A BEAUTIFUL VIEW OF DONNER LAKE.

GPS TRAILHEAD COORDINATES: N39° 18.870′ W120° 19.614′

DISTANCE & CONFIGURATION: 11.4-mile balloon loop

HIKING TIME: 3.5 hours

OUTSTANDING FEATURES: Views over Donner Lake and Shallenberger Ridge;
vistas from Castle Peak to Anderson Peak

ELEVATION: 7,051′ at trailhead

ACCESS: Year-round

MAPS: *Lake Tahoe Basin* (Trails Illustrated 803)

FACILITIES: Pit toilet

CONTACT: Tahoe National Forest, Truckee Ranger District, 530-587-3558,
www.fs.usda.gov/tahoe

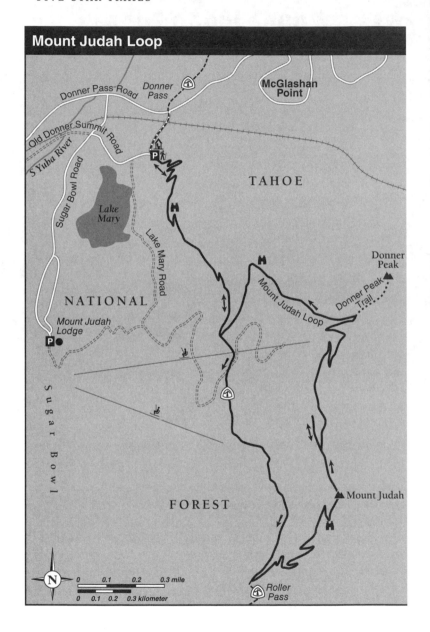

Mount Judah Loop

Donner Pass Road

Donner Pass Road

Donner Pass

McGlashan Point

Old Donner Summit Road

S Yuba River

Sugar Bowl Road

Lake Mary

Lake Mary Road

TAHOE

Donner Peak

Mount Judah Loop

Donner Peak Trail

NATIONAL

Mount Judah Lodge

Sugar Bowl

FOREST

Mount Judah

Roller Pass

N

0   0.1   0.2   0.3 mile

0   0.1   0.2   0.3 kilometer

Overview

Mount Judah is one of those rare attractions that seem to have it all for a quick adventure fix: a trailhead conveniently close to the highway; a well-tended trail that is only moderately difficult; beautiful vistas of the lakes, mountains, and wilderness terrain; and very little backtracking.

Your route takes you 2.6 miles from the trailhead to the summit, gaining nearly 1,200 feet in elevation.

Route Details

After making your way from the parking area to the trailhead, take time to look over the trailhead kiosk. Walking along the combined Pacific Crest Trail (PCT) and Overland Emigrant Trail, you'll be heading generally south for the first half of your trek. This is a moderate hike, but don't let its short length fool you. To stay adequately hydrated, you should carry at least 2 liters of water.

Leave the rocky trailhead and walk about 200 feet east under the cover of conifers. In about 200 feet, you will begin the first of seven switchbacks that help you gain 200 feet to the nose of this ridge above Lake Mary. From the easternmost point of the second switchback, you have a good vista of Donner Pass and the railroad tracks beneath it.

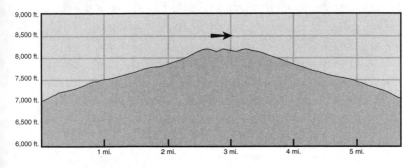

The trail remains quite rocky as the soils here are undeveloped and somewhat scarce.

The end of your switchbacks will bring you across to the west side of this ridge, traversing from north to south along the margin of this lightly forested slope. As you approach a chairlift visible above the ski runs ahead, be on the lookout for a junction with a trail to the east; this is where your loop will rejoin the PCT in another couple of hours.

In another 100 feet, look for a PCT sign posted up in a tree. As you clear the trees, you'll see a chairlift station above you to the east. Once you're directly under the chairlift, you're less than 500 feet from Lake Mary Road. Cross the road and pass one more chairlift station on your way north toward Roller Pass.

Located in the saddle between Mount Judah and Mount Lincoln, Roller Pass is marked by a rail anchored in the rock. It was named by Nicholas Carriger, a member of the original Donner party. He commented that, in September 1846, "we made a roller and fastened chains together and pulled wagons up with 12 yoke oxen on the top and the same at the bottom." Glance east for a quick appreciation of the ordeals they endured even before the snows arrived.

Retrace your steps a few hundred feet to the junction with the Mount Judah Loop, which heads uphill to the northeast. A reminder that no bicycles are allowed is attached to the trail sign. Parallel your trail for 550 feet before some short, easy switchbacks help you ascend through the trees. From this spot on the southeast end of the ridge, you will climb three sets of switchbacks (two S's and one Z) before reaching the summit.

As you wind your way up, you'll notice the frail, clinging vegetation—the pioneer species—that is also responsible for the soil-building you see in process. Pass by some scarily impressive volcanic "bombs" as you make your way. You'll see more of these massive conglomerates when you leave the summit, which is littered with smaller volcanic debris. Mount Judah's humble summit offers all hikers a well-deserved reward for their uphill efforts. The vista here is 360 degrees and does not disappoint. You can see the PCT as it disappears toward Anderson Peak, or gaze from Mount Lincoln to Mount Disney to Lake Van Norden, and even to Castle Peak. Views down to Donner Lake and Shallenberger Ridge can't be beaten.

The route north is obvious as it sticks to the spine of the ridge for the first 0.25 mile, then begins dipping below to the fir and hemlock of the east slope. Just before it dips downhill, you may notice a side trail angling off along the ridge to what looks like another peak. There is a trail, but it becomes indistinct at the north end and doesn't present an obvious route to rejoin this trail. Stay just beneath the ridgeline for another 0.25 mile where, under the microwave antennas, you descend two easy sets of switchbacks. Follow the track down to a junction with the trail leading off to the right to Donner Peak. A short hike of 0.25 mile gets you on top of that summit. The described hike leads to the left on a tired and faded Lake Mary Road. Follow this route by turning left on the Mount Judah Loop trail, which follows Lake Mary Road, which leads, more or less discernibly, for about 0.4 mile before the trail leaves the road and turns to the southwest. In about 0.25 mile, you'll intersect the PCT again. Turn north and retrace your steps to the trailhead.

Directions

Heading east on I-80, exit at Soda Springs and bear right on Donner Pass Road. Drive 3.6 miles and turn right. As you approach this turn, you'll see the Sugar Bowl gondola on the right and Donner Ski Ranch on the left. Turn at the next street to the right, Mount Judah Road, signed SUGAR BOWL–MOUNT JUDAH PARKING If you're coming from Truckee, take the Donner Pass Road exit from I-80 West and drive 7.1 miles to the SUGAR BOWL–MOUNT JUDAH PARKING sign on the left. Drive 0.15 mile and take the first left turn onto Old Donner Summit Road. Follow the road 0.15 mile to the small parking lot on the left, which has room for about 20 cars. The trailhead is 250 feet up the road on the right. There is a pit toilet at the trailhead parking lot.

39

Donner Pass to Squaw Valley

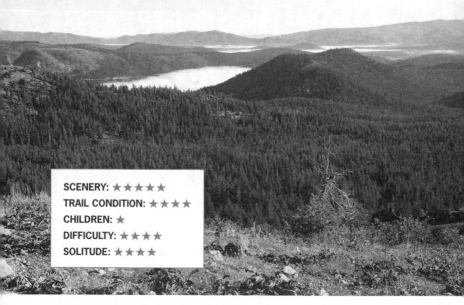

SCENERY: ★ ★ ★ ★ ★
TRAIL CONDITION: ★ ★ ★ ★
CHILDREN: ★
DIFFICULTY: ★ ★ ★ ★
SOLITUDE: ★ ★ ★ ★

NEAR ROLLER PASS, FOG DRAPES DONNER AND SEVERAL SMALLER LAKES.

GPS TRAILHEAD COORDINATES: N39° 18.868′ W120° 19.612′ (Donner Pass), N39° 11.968′ W120° 14.344′ (Squaw Valley–Granite Chief)

DISTANCE & CONFIGURATION: 15-mile point-to-point with shuttle

HIKING TIME: 9 hours

OUTSTANDING FEATURES: Incredible vistas, including the Royal Gorge of the North Fork of the American River; glacially smoothed and polished granite; fragmented and scorched volcanic debris; alpine meadows full of mule´s ears and ringed by fir trees draped with pale-green wolf lichen

ELEVATION: 7,051´ at trailhead

ACCESS: Year-round

MAPS: *Lake Tahoe Basin* (Trails Illustrated 803)

FACILITIES: Pit toilet

CONTACT: Tahoe National Forest, Truckee Ranger District, 530-587-3558, www.fs.usda.gov/tahoe

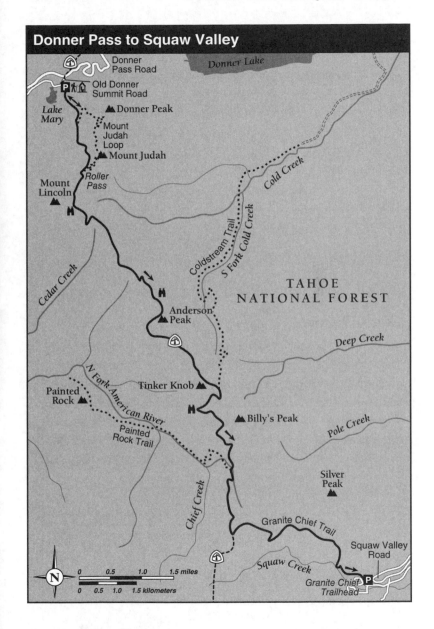

Donner Pass to Squaw Valley

Donner Pass Road
Old Donner Summit Road
Donner Lake
Lake Mary
Donner Peak
Mount Judah Loop
Mount Judah
Roller Pass
Mount Lincoln
Cold Creek
Cedar Creek
Coldstream Trail
S Fork Cold Creek
TAHOE NATIONAL FOREST
Anderson Peak
Deep Creek
N Fork American River
Painted Rock
Tinker Knob
Painted Rock Trail
Billy's Peak
Pole Creek
Silver Peak
Chief Creek
Granite Chief Trail
Squaw Valley Road
Squaw Creek
Granite Chief Trailhead

N

0   0.5   1.0   1.5 miles
0   0.5   1.0   1.5 kilometers

Overview

The Pacific Crest Trail (PCT) stretches 2,669 miles from Mexico to Canada. The terrain it covers between Donner Pass and Squaw Valley is among the most beautiful of the journey. Here, where the Sierra begins its slow descent for northbound hikers, southbound day hikers enjoy the reciprocal, an easy ascent into the backcountry. An uphill hike across forested ski slopes leads past Donner and Judah before crossing Roller Pass. Western hemlocks block the wind before you reach the apex of another exposed ridgeline, which you will follow to Anderson and on to Tinker. Descend into the upper reaches of the North Fork of the American River canyon, then traverse beneath Billy's Peak. Once across the headwaters of the North Fork, a 500-foot climb toward Granite Chief brings you to the trail descending to Squaw Valley, where you emerge next to the fire station.

Route Details

Check the information kiosk at the shared PCT–Overland Emigrant Trail trailhead. The map will give you an overview of the trails' relative locations and distances of the Tahoe National Forest north and south of Interstate I-80. Note that the only means of travel on the PCT is by foot or on horseback. Watch your step on the rocks and roots gracing the trail until the roots are replaced by switchbacks. Here your views will alternate between Donner Lake and Lake Mary. A brief hike up the nose of this ridge leads to a traverse of its western slope.

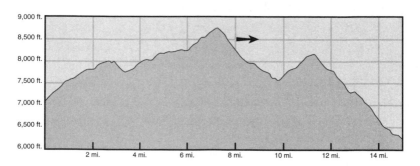

In about 1 mile, you'll reach the northern junction of the Mount Judah Loop trail and the PCT. Continue toward the chairlift on the left and past the snow-making apparatus. Note the PCT emblems attached to trees on the right. Walk past a beautiful meadow (terrain park) and presently cross Lake Mary Road, where a sign on the red fir reminds bikers not to be here.

Continue hiking south, in and out of trees and on and off of the rock of Mount Judah's slopes. As you veer slightly southwest, after little more than an hour on the trail you'll find the marker for the south end of the Mount Judah Ridge. Here, you'll have an excellent vista down into Sugar Bowl. Historic Roller Pass commemorates part of the Donner party, who persevered in bringing their wagons over this spot in September 1846 by laying rails and yoking oxen to their wagons to haul them over this rounded saddle.

Continue on to the right and uphill through hemlock, south-bound on the east flank of Mount Lincoln toward the distant ridge. Just before you emerge from the hemlocks, you'll see a possible bivy site on the downhill side of the trail.

Once you make it out onto the ridge, you'll be exposed to some ferocious gusts, evidenced by the scant vegetation and clean-swept trail. You will stay on this ridge for about the next 2.75 miles. A con-veniently located signpost declares that Anderson Peak is 4 miles south, and Tinker Knob, an additional 2 miles. Put your head down so the wind glides by and trudge onward.

Vistas to the north now include Mount Judah and Castle Peak. The trail flanks the eroding east slope of Mount Lincoln, where bound-ary signs warn skiers away from the cliffs. Views to the south include Anderson Peak and Tinker Knob. Vistas to the east include Donner Lake and Shallenberger Ridge. Before you enter the trees again, you can see your trail ahead quite distinctly against the near-naked terrain.

The trail is quite exposed on the left, but if you're here in the fall, you may not notice it for the sound made by the profusion of woolly mule's ears. Fuzzy and silent and forming a sea of yellow in the summer, early fall sees them dry and brown, creating a wind song of rustling and rattling leaves. Regardless of their seasonal beauty, they make an ineffective windbreak. Two gentle switchbacks send you downhill briefly through the trees before gaining the ridge again.

Your vistas to the west are magnificent across this landscape of thin and gravelly soils held down by intermittent swaths of conifers that alternate with vast, sloping meadows of mule's ears and lupine. Leave the Western white pine and red fir to cross the ridge on the way to Anderson Peak. To the east is a good deal of exposed trail with sharp drop-offs.

A couple of switchbacks will help you up the next rounded hill before you continue an easy uphill traverse to Anderson Peak. At the next trail junction near the foot of that peak, leave the rustling mule's ears and golden buckwheat behind, and follow the PCT as it heads west, to the right. A blocked trail to Benson Hut continues south, uphill straight ahead. Continue past and, as you head to the southwest on this forested slope, a new trail to Benson Hut intersects the PCT at a trail sign directly below the summit.

Your course now is to continue—with broken pieces of mountain above you, below you, and under your feet—navigating around decaying Anderson Peak before resuming your southward course about 0.5 mile along the ridgeline toward Tinker Knob. Your path will be interrupted by a sign, decorated with a historic PCT emblem, that confirms the name of this crumbling roadblock that you're rounding and indicates a 4-mile hike back to Mount Lincoln.

Your path follows the windswept ridgeline to Tinker Knob, where it follows the undulating terrain uphill to a junction with the summit trail, which is set squarely in the middle of the North Slope. Follow the PCT by staying to the left; a sign with Tinker's name and elevation is just 100 yards away.

Descend to the southeast across a broad slope filled with mule's ears and interrupted only by an occasional fir. Your vista to the southwest is one captured from this spot alone: a view into the Royal Gorge—the North Fork of the American River Canyon. Descending through the mule's ears to the junction just ahead brings you to the

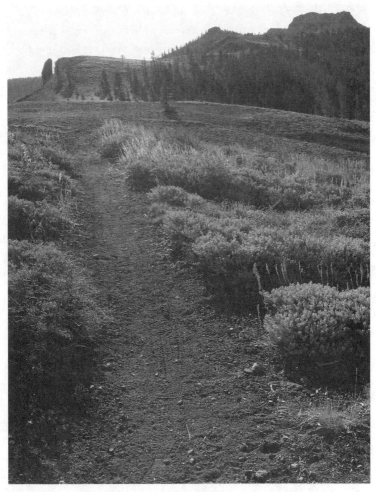

THE PCT IS CLOSED TO WHEELED VEHICLES—TRACKS ARE MADE BY SCOFFLAWS.

eastern edge of this ridge for the last time. A sharp left turn would put you on the Coldstream Trail, which would deliver you 7 miles away to Truckee.

Follow the PCT as it traverses along this margin past a PCT signpost. In about 200 yards, 7.5 miles from your trailhead, begin descending a total of 1,050 feet to the headwaters of the North Fork of the American River. Start a businesslike descent on a southerly switchback, and take a U-turn back to the north before a long, undulating switchback down to about 8,100 feet, where you will get a different but still excellent vista into the Royal Gorge. Here, you'll make an abrupt turn to the east, beginning a long, loopy traverse beneath Billy's Peak. Be on the lookout for a year-round spring 0.25 mile ahead. A second spring feeds the creek that you'll cross in another 100 yards. About 300 yards after that you'll spot a suitable campsite in the flat spot a few hundred feet off the trail, sheltered by a copse of conifers.

Descend to the south, and shortly after emerging from the trees, enter another field of mule's ears sitting on top of volcanic soil with several runoff drainages. The area also supports a proliferation of firs, which easily take root here. Just before crossing another runoff stream in the apex of this canyon, you will find late-blooming clarkia along with Indian rhubarb and tobacco brush. Cross the stream and head uphill into the Western white pines and red firs. Just before the ascent, note a suitable bivy site on the east side of the trail. In a few hundred feet another broad vista opens up to the west for you.

Continue descending next to this huge granite wall, your trail graced by Jeffrey pine and Western juniper. If you notice a subliminal craving for butterscotch at this time, blame it on the Jeffrey pines, which emit a butterscotch or vanilla scent from their bark. As the PCT crosses bare granite slopes, follow the ducks (rock trail markers) or, in some places, the faint blue or red blazes painted on trailside boulders. When you come upon a fractured PCT sign and a seasonal stream, look for good bivy sites near a large meadow about 200 yards to the southeast. In less than 200 feet, you'll come upon the Painted Rock Trail, which heads to the northwest. From here, about 10 miles from your trailhead, you'll begin a 650-foot ascent to the Granite Chief Trail, just 1.1 miles ahead.

As a side trip from this point, look for the trail about 1,000 feet ahead on the left, which leads up to Mountain Meadow Lake. The unmaintained trail parallels the PCT and meets the PCT at the Granite Chief Trail junction 1.2 miles ahead, so no backtracking would be necessary if you wanted to take that route. On the PCT, ascend the ridge via two sets of Z-shaped switchbacks, and continue along the ridge until you fall away to the right to skirt this knob above you. Stay just below the ridge until you reach the PCT signpost. Ten paces farther south is the junction of the Granite Chief Trail. If you wanted to bag another peak, it's only 1.5 miles from that junction to Granite Chief's peak.

The described trail turns northeast and begins descending the 4 miles to Squaw Valley. In another 500 feet, you get a momentary view of Lake Tahoe in the distance. Descend through the forest on five switchbacks, which are interrupted by a small meadow. Continue losing elevation as you travel east at the foot of Silver Peak's smaller companion. As you approach a much larger alpine meadow, notice the blaze in the shape of the small letter *i* on the solitary white pine surrounded by firs. The trail is rather rocky now as it heads through sagebrush and buckbrush into the aspens.

As soon as you hit the polished granite, your destination comes into view. Decay seems to be the word of the moment on this slope. Fallen trees left in place over decades have left their mark on the rock, which is itself splitting, shattering, and crumbling. Follow the ducks past mountain pride penstemon occupying cracks and crevices, soil-packed refuges for seeds. While the trail is easy to follow, pay close attention as it descends at a fair pace. Remember to look for ducks and now gold- or yellow-painted blazes. Three short legs will navigate you around an obstacle near the top of this outcrop—500 feet west, 200 feet south, and 500 feet east—before you descend into a glacially carved ravine. Your trail across the canyon comes into view and you descend slowly northeast toward the far canyon wall generally clinging to the north wall.

Your path is a gentle and quiet descent well above Squaw Creek. You have about 700 feet left to descend; look for a spring on the uphill side of the trail while you're still traveling east. Indian paintbrush is a constant trailside partner as you cross small streams about four times over the next 0.5 mile. Follow the ducks closely, and continue heading slightly southeast over the next 150 vertical feet down to the trailhead. The trail terminates at the sign next to the fire station in Squaw Valley.

Directions

Heading east on I-80, exit at Soda Springs and bear right on Donner Pass Road. Drive 3.6 miles and turn right. As you approach this turn, you'll see the Sugar Bowl gondola on the right and Donner Ski Ranch on the left. Turn at the next street to the right, Mount Judah Road, signed SUGAR BOWL–MOUNT JUDAH PARKING. If you're coming from Truckee, take the Donner Pass Road exit from I-80 West, and drive 7.1 miles to the SUGAR BOWL–MOUNT JUDAH PARKING sign on the left. Drive 0.15 mile, and take the first left turn onto Old Donner Summit Road. Follow the road 0.15 mile to the small parking lot on the left, which has room for about 20 cars. The trailhead is 250 feet up the road on the right. There is a pit toilet at the trailhead parking lot.

You'll also need to leave a shuttle vehicle at Squaw Valley. From Truckee, drive about 12 miles south on CA 89 toward Tahoe City. At the light, turn right onto Squaw Valley Road. Bear right at the Y (Squaw Ridge Road), and continue on Squaw Valley Road about 1.75 miles to Olympic Village. The signed trailhead is on the east side of the fire station; another trail access stands 200 yards to the west, at a small parking area on the north side of the Olympic Village Inn.

To reach Squaw Valley from South Lake Tahoe, drive west on US 50 (Lake Tahoe Boulevard) 2.4 miles to CA 89 North (Emerald Bay Road). Turn right and drive about 27.5 miles north to the Y in Tahoe City. Turn left and continue about 5.5 miles on CA 89 North to the light at Squaw Valley Road. Turn left to continue toward the Olympic Village and the trailhead.

40 # Loch Leven Lakes

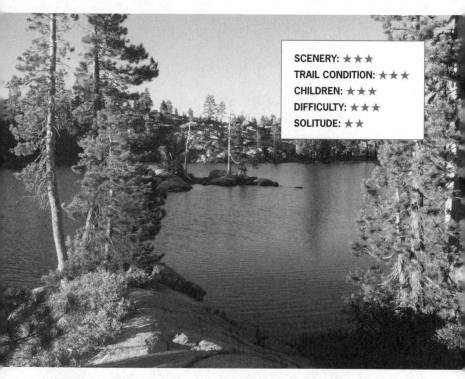

HIGH LOCH LEVEN LAKE OFFERS SOME COMFORTABLE CAMPSITES.

SCENERY: ★ ★ ★
TRAIL CONDITION: ★ ★ ★
CHILDREN: ★ ★ ★
DIFFICULTY: ★ ★ ★
SOLITUDE: ★ ★

GPS TRAILHEAD COORDINATES: N39° 18.559′ W120° 30.854′

DISTANCE & CONFIGURATION: 6.6–8.2-mile out-and-back

HIKING TIME: 4 hours

OUTSTANDING FEATURES: Three subalpine lakes within easy reach of the trailhead, which is conveniently located close to Big Bend west of Donner Summit

ELEVATION: 5,761′ at trailhead

ACCESS: Year-round

MAPS: *Tahoe National Forest West* (Trails Illustrated 804)

FACILITIES: Pit toilet

CONTACT: Tahoe National Forest, Big Bend Visitor Center, 530-426-3609, www.fs.usda.gov/tahoe

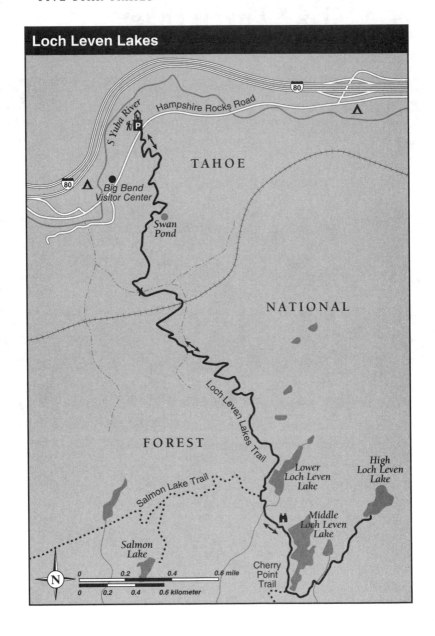

Loch Leven Lakes

80

Hampshire Rocks Road

S Yuba River

P

TAHOE

80

Big Bend
Visitor Center

Swan
Pond

NATIONAL

Loch Leven Lakes Trail

FOREST

Salmon Lake Trail

High
Loch Leven
Lake

Lower
Loch Leven
Lake

Middle
Loch Leven
Lake

Salmon
Lake

Cherry
Point
Trail

N

| 0 | 0.2 | 0.4 | 0.6 mile |
| 0 | 0.2 | 0.4 | 0.6 kilometer |

Overview

Loch Leven's convenient trailhead access makes this a popular day-hike destination. Hikers are rewarded for their 1,000-foot uphill climb with a selection of subalpine lakes and generous vistas of tree-clad and exposed-granite slopes festooned with flowers of every color.

Route Details

Your hike to Loch Leven Lakes begins at about 5,800 feet in elevation on the south side of Hampshire Rocks Road. While you will navigate generally southeast, you'll need to pay close attention to the obvious trail, often marked by ducks (rock trail markers), as it winds around some of the granite outcrops that characterize this terrain. Initially, rocky switchbacks will help you gain a bit of elevation above the road. It seems as if each crack and crevice in every granite step is graced by penstemon in early July. The flat, sandy, gravelly spots are decorated with pale-pink pussytoes. And there's more color to come.

The trail follows the terrain back to the east, crossing a marshy area before ascending on granite-block steps to the west. More switchbacks and changes of direction will bring you up a boulder staircase along a granite slab that ends beneath a large juniper. Ducks will line your path and may sit on top of boulders that form your trail

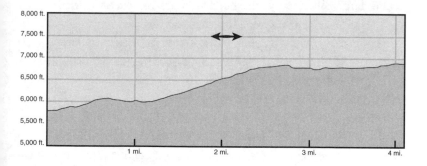

across the granite, leading to a copse of lodgepole pines and a small granite dome on the trail's north side.

A small runoff pond, just large enough to attract a squadron of mosquitoes, crowds the trail as you head west outlining the edge of this rounded granite block. In a moment, you will spy railroad tracks off to the west at the point where they emerge from the tunnels originally built by Chinese laborers for the Central Pacific Railroad. Head south and descend toward the creek, where you will cross on a footbridge that attracts radiant orange and red columbine. From the footbridge, 1 mile from the trailhead, you will make a short, traversing ascent east to the railroad tracks 0.25 mile away.

The trail reaches the tracks beneath the signal light structure. Across the tracks sits a control box right next to your trail. Cross the double tracks here, and resume ascending the trail. Please exercise caution: If you can see a train just as it emerges from the tunnels, you'll probably arrive at the track junction at the same time as the train. Trains run in both directions around the clock.

The first of a baker's dozen of switchbacks up your 800-foot climb begins by heading southwest. Intermittent sunshine breaks through the top of this fir forest, spotlighting the deep-purple larkspur, bright-red Indian paintbrush, subtle-blue lupine, and yellow wallflower. About 1.4 miles past the railroad tracks, you will notice the sun shining on you more brightly as the trees thin out and the terrain contours more to reach a notch overlooking lake number one.

Descend on the rocky trail to a small clearing adjacent to Lower Loch Leven Lake, where a sign informs: MIDDLE LOCH LEVEN LAKE— 0.25 MILE, CHERRY POINT TRAIL—0.5 MILE, HIGH LOCH LEVEN LAKE—1 MILE. The trail at the end of the first lake leads southwest to Salmon Lake, just about a mile away.

It's only a short walk to picturesque Loch Leven's middle lake, where checkerspot and hairstreak butterflies are dizzily mauling the heather. The lake has small beaches to lounge on, islands to swim out to, and some nice campsites. The trail at the south end of the middle lake leads to the North Fork of the American River, 8 miles distant, along the Big Granite Trail.

More solitude and secluded bivy spots can be found when you ascend just about 250 feet over a fast, granite-filled 0.6 mile to High Loch Leven Lake. The vistas enlarge along with the granite boulders and slabs. Enjoy an off-season overnight here or a fun anytime day hike. Fill up on fresh air here and have fun on the way back to the trailhead.

Directions

Heading east on I-80 from Sacramento, take Exit 166 to Big Bend. In 0.3 mile, turn left on Hampshire Rocks Road, and drive 0.4 mile to a parking area on the north side of the road.

Heading west on I-80 from Reno, take Exit 168 toward Big Bend/Rainbow Road, and turn left toward Hampshire Rocks Road. Make a slight right onto Hampshire Rocks Road and drive 0.9 mile to the trailhead parking.

Pit toilets are available at this popular parking area. The signed trailhead is on the south side of the road, across from the parking area.

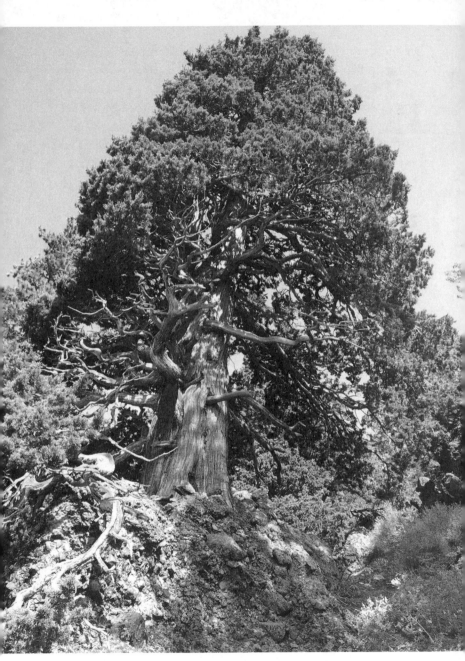

WESTERN JUNIPER WORKS HARD TO TURN VOLCANIC ROCK INTO FRIABLE SOIL.

Appendix A: Managing Agencies

Eldorado National Forest
www.fs.usda.gov/eldorado
100 Forni Road, Placerville, CA 95667
530-622-5061

AMADOR RANGER DISTRICT
26820 Silver Drive, Pioneer, CA 95666
209-295-4251

Humboldt-Toiyabe National Forest
www.fs.usda.gov/htnf
1200 Franklin Way, Sparks, NV 89431
775-331-6444

CARSON RANGER DISTRICT
1536 S. Carson St., Carson City, NV 89701
775-882-2766

Lake Tahoe Nevada State Park
parks.nv.gov/parks/marlette-hobart-backcountry
PO Box 6116, Incline Village, NV 89452
775-831-0494

Tahoe National Forest
www.fs.usda.gov/tahoe
631 Coyote St., Nevada City, CA 95959
530-265-453

BIG BEND VISITOR CENTER
49685 Hampshire Rocks Road (Old US 40)
(at the I-80 exits for Big Bend or Rainbow Road)
PO Box 830, Soda Springs, CA 95728
530-426-3609

TRUCKEE RANGER DISTRICT
(Donner Pass, Little Truckee Summit, Truckee River/CA 89 South, NV 267 areas)
10811 Stockrest Springs Road, Truckee, CA 96161
530-587-3558

(continued)

Tahoe Rim Trail Association

tahoerimtrail.org
128 Market St., Suite 3E, Stateline, NV 89449
775-298-4485

US Forest Service, Lake Tahoe Basin Management Unit

www.fs.usda.gov/ltbmu
35 College Drive, South Lake Tahoe, CA 96150
530-543-2600

NORTH SHORE OFFICE

855 Alder Ave., Incline Village, NV 89450
775-831-0914

TAYLOR CREEK VISITOR CENTER

tinyurl.com/taylorcreekvisitorcenter
About 3 miles north of South Lake Tahoe, on the lake side of CA 89
530-543-2674

Appendix B: Permits

California Campfire Permit

You must have a campfire permit to use a stove, lantern, charcoal grill, or wood campfire outside of a developed campground or recreation area in California. The permit is your agreement to follow the campfire restrictions and regulations in effect. Go to preventwildfireca.org/campfire-permit to fill out an application form.

Wilderness Permits

Eldorado National Forest cooperatively manages two wilderness areas with Humboldt-Toiyabe and Stanislaus National Forests and the Lake Tahoe Basin Management Unit. Both **Desolation Wilderness** and **Mokelumne Wilderness** require permits year-round for overnight stays; Desolation Wilderness also requires day permits.

Permit requirements and processes differ significantly between the two; to learn more about these wilderness areas and to find out how to acquire permits for them, check out www.fs.usda.gov/main/eldorado/passes-permits/recreation.

Pick up permits to enter the west side of Desolation Wilderness at the **Pacific Ranger District** office (530-644-6048; call for seasonal hours), located on 7887 CA 50, 4 miles east of Pollock Pines near Fresh Pond.

Pick up permits to enter the east side of Desolation Wilderness at the **Taylor Creek Visitor Center** (530-543-2674, open May–October; call for hours), located on CA 89, 3 miles north of the CA 50/CA 89 junction in South Lake Tahoe, or the **Lake Tahoe Basin Management Unit** (530-543-2600; open weekdays, 8 a.m.–4:30 p.m.), located at 35 College Drive, 2 miles east of the CA 50/CA 89 junction in South Lake Tahoe. From CA 50, turn right on Al Tahoe Boulevard, then turn right at the first signal.

Pick up permits to enter Mokelumne Wilderness (except for the Carson Pass Management Area—see next section) at the **Amador Ranger District** office (209-295-4251; call for seasonal hours), just off CA 88 at 26820 Silver Drive in Pioneer, and the **Carson Pass Information Station** (209-258-8606, open summer only; call for hours), on CA 88 at the summit of Carson Pass.

The best way to obtain an overnight camping permit in either area is to use the online service **Recreation.gov.** There is a $6 fee for the permit, plus the fee for overnight camping. The convenience of this service cannot be overstated.

CARSON PASS MANAGEMENT AREA   Because of the popularity of this special area within Mokelumne Wilderness, restrictions are in effect to ensure your opportunities for solitude and a primitive recreational experience, and to protect popular camping destinations from overcrowding and heavy impacts. See the details at tinyurl.com/carsonpass.

Whereas the national forests mostly cooperate in their management practices regarding Desolation and Mokelumne Wildernesses, Carson Pass is a notable exception. The Amador Ranger District office, in Eldorado National Forest, cannot issue permits for this area, even though part of Mokelumne Wilderness is in the same forest; permits can be obtained only at the **Carson Pass Information Station** (see above), in Humboldt-Toiyabe National Forest. Other cases like this exist, so always call ahead to clarify the current permit situation.

Forest Annual Day Use Pass

This pass allows you to park at several popular trailhead facilities in Desolation and Mokelumne Wildernesses, including **Eagle Falls, Pyramid Creek, Carson Pass, Carson Overflow,** and **Meiss Parking Areas.** (Eagle Falls and Pyramid Creek waive day-use fees for holders of overnight permits.)

The pass is not exactly annual, though. There is a summer pass and a Sno-Park pass; the dates are roughly May–November for one and November–May for the other. The pass costs $25—with day-use parking normally $5 a day, it offers a big savings if you intend to do more than one overnight trip in the specific areas above. The passes are available at the **Taylor Creek Visitor Center** (530-543-2674) and the **Carson Pass Information Station** (209-258-8606); some local businesses also sell them.

 # Appendix C: Maps

Maps are an essential piece of gear that may play a vital role in your safety on even the tamest day hike.

I carried these waterproof maps with me on every hike, and their condition after more than 40 hikes shows their utility and durability.

Desolation Wilderness and the South Lake Tahoe Basin Recreation Map. Birmingham, AL: Wilderness Press, 2015.

A Guide to the Desolation Wilderness. Eldorado National Forest and Lake Tahoe Basin Management Unit. San Francisco: US Forest Service, Pacific Southwest Region, 2000.

Lake Tahoe Basin Trail Map. Adventure Maps Inc., 2011.

Lake Tahoe Basin (US Forest Service), California/Nevada. Trails Illustrated Map 803. Evergreen, CO: National Geographic Maps, 2006.

Lake Tahoe Recreation Map: Tahoe Rim Trail. San Rafael, CA: Tom Harrison Maps, 2007.

Tahoe National Forest East (Sierra Buttes, Donner Pass), California. Trails Illustrated Map 805. Evergreen, CO: National Geographic Maps, 2006.

Tahoe National Forest West (Yuba and American Rivers), California. Trails Illustrated Map 804. Evergreen, CO: National Geographic Maps, 2006.

Mokelumne Wilderness. US Forest Service, Pacific Southwest Region. San Francisco, CA: 1987.

Appendix D:
Suggested Reading

Arno, Stephen F. *Discovering Sierra Trees*. Yosemite, CA: Yosemite Association, 1973.

Basey, Harold E. *Discovering Sierra Reptiles and Amphibians*. Yosemite, CA: Yosemite Association, 2004.

Blackwell, Laird R. *Wildflowers of the Sierra Nevada and the Central Valley*. Edmonton, AB, Canada: Lone Pine Press, 1999.

Blackwell, Laird R., *Tahoe Wildflowers: A Month-by-Month Guide to Wildflowers in the Tahoe Basin and Surrounding Areas*. Helena, MT: A Falcon Guide, 2007.

Hill, Mary. *Geology of the Sierra Nevada*. Berkeley: University of California Press, 2006.

Horn, Elizabeth L. *Sierra Nevada Wildflowers*. Missoula, MT: Mountain Press Company, 1998.

James, George Wharton. *The Lake of the Sky—Lake Tahoe*. Boston: L. C. Page & Company, 1915.

Laws, John Muir. *The Laws Field Guide to the Sierra Nevada*. Berkeley: Heyday Books, 2007.

Lekish, Barbara. *Tahoe Place Names*. Lafayette, CA: Great West Books, 1988.

Miller, Millie, and Cyndi Nelson. *Talons: North American Birds of Prey*. Boulder, CO: Johnson Books, 1989.

Murie, Olaus J. *Peterson Field Guide: A Field Guide to Animal Tracks*. Boston: Houghton Mifflin Company, 1974.

Niehaus, Theodore F., and Charles L. Ripper. *Peterson Field Guide: A Field Guide to Pacific States Wildflowers*. Boston: Houghton Mifflin Company, 1976.

Powers, Phil. *National Outdoor Leadership School Wilderness Mountaineering*. Mechanicsburg, PA: Stackpole Books, 1993.

Russo, Ron, and Pam Olhausan. *Mammal Finder.* Berkeley: Nature Study Guild, 1987.

Schimelpfenig, Todd, and Linda Lindsey. *National Outdoor Leadership School Wilderness First Aid,* 3rd ed. Mechanicsburg, PA: Stackpole Books, 2000.

Storer, Tracy I., Robert L. Usinger, and David Lukas. *Sierra Nevada Natural History.* Berkeley: University of California Press, 2004.

Thomas, John H., and Dennis R. Parnell. *Native Shrubs of the Sierra Nevada.* Berkeley: University of California Press, 1974.

Underhill, J. E. *Sagebrush Wildflowers.* Blaine, WA: Hancock House, Inc., 1986.

Wells, Darran. *National Outdoor Leadership School Wilderness Navigation.* Mechanicsburg, PA: Stackpole Books, 2005.

Whitman, Ann H., ed. *Audubon Society Guide: Familiar Trees of North America: Western Region.* New York: Alfred A. Knopf, 1988.

Whitney, Stephen. *A Sierra Club Naturalist's Guide: The Sierra Nevada.* San Francisco: Sierra Club Books, 1979.

Index

Page references followed by *m* indicate a map.

About the Author

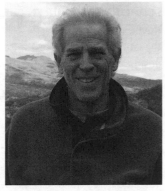

Photo: Karin Connolly

JORDAN SUMMERS has had more fun camping on rock, dirt, and snow than should be allowed. Hiking has been his go-to escape route for way too many years. To put it bluntly, he has gone from being an ultra-heavy hiker to a nearly lightweight one. (Some skills just take time, but losing the gear weight is essential.)

Jordan is a volunteer for the Pacific Crest Trail Association and the Tahoe Rim Trail Association. Whether it's building trail, guiding hikers, training guides, or just yakking out loud about where to go and how to come back, Jordan is all in.

His passion: to turn on hiking neophytes to get out there, to have fun while they're out there, to respect what's out there, and to come home safely from there.

DEAR CUSTOMERS AND FRIENDS,

SUPPORTING YOUR INTEREST IN OUTDOOR ADVENTURE, travel, and an active lifestyle is central to our operations, from the authors we choose to the locations we detail to the way we design our books. Menasha Ridge Press was incorporated in 1982 by a group of veteran outdoorsmen and professional outfitters. For many years now, we've specialized in creating books that benefit the outdoors enthusiast.

Almost immediately, Menasha Ridge Press earned a reputation for revolutionizing outdoors- and travel-guidebook publishing. For such activities as canoeing, kayaking, hiking, backpacking, and mountain biking, we established new standards of quality that transformed the whole genre, resulting in outdoor-recreation guides of great sophistication and solid content. Menasha Ridge Press continues to be outdoor publishing's greatest innovator.

The folks at Menasha Ridge Press are as at home on a whitewater river or mountain trail as they are editing a manuscript. The books we build for you are the best they can be, because we're responding to your needs. Plus, we use and depend on them ourselves.

We look forward to seeing you on the river or the trail. If you'd like to contact us directly, visit us at menasharidge.com. We thank you for your interest in our books and the natural world around us all.

SAFE TRAVELS,

Bob Sehlinger

BOB SEHLINGER
PUBLISHER